When I last met Slim in October of 2005, he showed me and a friend of mine his shop where he made his wondrous Light-Life Tools. I have had good experiences with his tools, especially the Acu-Vac Coil. It has positive health effects and seems to stimulate the pineal gland by eliciting vivid dreams when I put it underneath my pillow. Slim's Light-Life Tools produce a flow of subtle energies, a primordial form of force or energy, which must be primary to our known forces in physics, yet to be discovered by science.

Stephan Fuelling, Ph.D. Physicist

T0147418

* * *

Slim in action was irresistible; to listen to him was spellbinding. I thought of him as Merlin, the Master of Energy. He introduced me to the quantum power of subtle energy and its role in my every moment. Working with his tools, I experienced miracle after miracle until I realized that was always Slim's point. Life is a miracle that we have the power and obligation to utilize. He gives us the tools and the wisdom to live life as it was designed. The truth and simplicity of the universe unfold in these pages as a guide to each of us, encouraging, loving, and like Slim, always fun.

Tana Blackmore, Founder of Sacred Ground International

* * *

As a friend and colleague of Slim Spurling's, I know his passion was to work toward healing Planet Earth and every living thing on it. His Light-Life Technology and techniques work! Susan Anderson enlightens us with both previously unwritten about and advanced technologies. A "must read" for those who wish to join in the healing of our planet *and* for your own enlightenment.

Judy Lavine, Medical Intuitive, Healer, Shaman

* * *

I had the privilege of working with Slim from 1993 until his passing in 2007. We had a common passion, the desire for knowledge gained by the personal experience of nature and the application of that knowledge providing the wisdom of the mystical quantum world. That wisdom, we found, was revealed over time from patience and a belief that nature would always reveal her secrets for those who had the ears to hear and the eyes to see. It was that faith that seemed to always provide the answers Slim was looking for. Many of our discussions over the years we worked together were based on practical application of the Light-Life™ Tools, and yet the personal and theoretical components of the reasons why the tools worked were based on the quantum rules, as best we understood them at the time, and the comparison of those rules with what we each learned from nature.

Randy Kemberling, Doctor of Chiropractic

* * *

The moment I was exposed to Slim Spurling's Harmonizers, I signed up for a workshop with Katharina Spurling-Kaffl, knowing I would ask a group of people to come on board to clean the air in Albany, New York. As a body worker and distributor of these magnificent tools, I have had the privilege of seeing everything from faster recovery from broken bones, inflammations, cuts, and burns ~ to people, including myself, making sweeping life changes. The tools support growth and change. I take them wherever I go, and the applications for their use continue to unfold.

Virginia Houck, LMT

IN THE MIND OF A MASTER

By Susan Anderson,
with Slim Spurling

iUniverse, Inc.
Bloomington

In the Mind of a Master

Light-Life™ is a trademark of IX-EL, Inc.
Editing by Diane Covington
Cover Design by KillerCovers.com
Photographs by Chris Kokias

iUniverse books may be ordered through booksellers or by contacting:

iUniverse
1663 Liberty Drive
Bloomington, IN 47403
www.iuniverse.com
1-800-Authors (1-800-288-4677)

ISBN: 978-1-4759-3072-6 (sc)
ISBN: 978-1-4759-3073-3 (hc)
ISBN: 978-1-4759-3074-0 (e)

Library of Congress Control Number: 2012910559

Printed in the United States of America

iUniverse rev. date: 8/21/2012

DISCLAIMER

The information in this book is designed to provide helpful information on the subjects discussed. This book is not meant to be used, nor should it be used, to diagnosis or treat any medical condition. For diagnosis or treatment of any medical problem, consult your own physician. Neither the publisher, nor the authors, nor Katharina Spurling-Kaffl, nor IX-EL, Inc. and their employees, nor their authorized distributors are responsible for any specific health or medical needs that may require medical supervision, and are not liable for any damages or negative consequences from any treatment, action, application, or preparation to any person reading or following the information in this book. Neither the publisher, nor the authors, nor Katharina Spurling-Kaffl, nor IX-EL, Inc. and their employees, nor their authorized distributors are responsible for any physical, psychological, emotional, financial, or commercial damages or negative consequences from any treatment or action to any person reading or following the information in this book.

No statement in the book, unless indicated, has been evaluated by the U.S. Food and Drug Administration. No product mentioned or alluded to is intended to diagnosis, treat, cure, or prevent any disease or other medical condition.

Expressed or implied warranties are disclaimed, including, but not limited to, warranties of merchantability, fitness for a particular purpose, accuracy and completeness, title or non-infringement. Information contained in this book is intended as an educational aid only, and is the opinion only of the authors and the experiences of those whose written testimonials are included.

The stated properties of the Light-Life™ Tools are founded in years of direct observation and close study. These products were developed by a team of research scientists and psychics for experimental research and educational purposes only. The information in this book is an attempt to inform the reader on the function and use of this technology. It is in no way meant to be taken as a statement of fact, but rather the opinion of the author, Slim Spurling, and Katharina Spurling-Kaffl that the Light-Life™ Tools work as so described. Neither the publisher, nor the authors, nor Katharina Spurling-Kaffl, nor IX-EL, Inc. and their employees, nor their authorized distributors accept any responsibility for how the reader chooses to apply this information or for the results that they obtain when they do. The healing techniques and methods described herein are based on up to 21 years of practical application and experience. They are meant to supplement, not to be a substitute for, professional medical care or treatment.

TABLE OF CONTENTS

FOREWORD

When I met Slim in September of 1997, it was like recognizing an old friend. For him, it was clear from the moment we met that something important was going to happen. We were in Germany, where Slim was teaching two workshops organized by my brother Michael Kaffl. I had been invited to translate and had prepared for the workshop by reading the workbook Slim and his partners had published. I was intrigued by his dowsing technique! Living in Bavaria, Germany, I was familiar with dowsing, as it is very common there. It has been practiced since the Middle Ages and even earlier. Käthe Bachler, an Austrian dowser, found geopathic stress contributed to Attention Deficit Disorder (ADD) and Sudden Infant Death Syndrome (SIDS), as well as many other ailments. Truly, it was and still is a worrisome issue.

Slim's genius was to find a remedy to block geopathic stress lines. The most common remedy German dowsers suggested when they found a water vein under your bed or any other interference, for example, the Hartmann Grid, was to move your furniture around to avoid those areas. Sleeping, standing, or sitting on an intersection of geopathic, Hartmann Grid, or other stress lines could cause, amongst other harms, lack of focus, ill health, or even death. Slim's technique was effective and simple to implement. I was hooked! To now have a remedy for geopathic stress-related issues was not all that excited me. When I discovered what the tools could do for people, agriculture, and the environment, I was really on fire! I knew I wanted to help spread the word. And mind you, at that time, Slim had only eight products: the ½, 1, and 3½ Sacred Cubit Rings; three Harmonizers in Sacred Cubit size – the Personal, Environmental, and Agricultural; the Acu-Vac Coil; and the Feedback Loop; all in 24K gold plated copper.

Well, long story short, we were married in May of 2001, and during our time together, we developed several new lines of products. Slim and I traveled frequently to conferences where he was a speaker, and to workshops people sponsored for him. At one of these workshops, in November 2006, I met Susan and Scott Anderson. Slim had met them previously in August at an event in New York City. I liked them right away and felt as though I had known them forever. Little did I expect they would soon play such an important role in my life. Today, I am happy to call both good friends.

On November 12, 2007, following a six-month illness, Slim passed from this physical earth plane. Slim's transition was a devastating loss for me. His departure was also deeply mourned by our staff, family, friends, and many people around the world who loved and respected him. We do appreciate that his spirit is still around and inspires my team and I. We have created many new items, all based on sacred geometry, and which are mentioned in this book. Our research and development of new products continues.

Slim passed on his legacy of the Light-Life™ Technology to me, as he trusted my integrity. He knew without question that I would continue with our work. When it was time to present the first workshop on Slim's dowsing and stress reduction technique and the introduction and application of the tools, I was looking for a good dowser who was familiar with Slim's work. Scott Anderson immediately came to mind as someone I was confident could teach dowsing, while keeping the integrity of Slim's techniques intact. To my good fortune, he agreed to teach dowsing at my workshops. Scott is like a brother to me, and always fun to be around. He is a Master Dowser, and Susan is very proficient in different types of dowsing, as well. Their vast knowledge of dowsing goes far beyond what we had time to teach in our workshops. Ultimately, we decided to offer an advanced class for people who wanted to delve deeper into the art of dowsing. Scott and Susan taught their first workshop together here in Colorado in 2010, and I was impressed by how well Susan had organized and structured their instructional materials.

When it was time for a new book to be written, Susan was the logical choice to author it. She knew the tools from her own experience, and it also helped that we have a good rapport and she could effectively put into proper American English what I wanted to convey. While writing this book was quite a test for Susan, finishing it – meaning adding my pieces of information – was also quite a challenge for me. Almost every day we get new field reports from people using the tools, and I'm like, oh, I want this in the book, this is so important for people to know. Then we create another tool, and that tool's description and purpose should be included, and so on. You get the picture, right?! So please understand that the information in this book is a work in progress. You will find continually updated information on our website **www.LightLifeTechnology.com**. Also, as we find new ways of using the 'old' tools, we will, of course, share that with you as well.

It was almost as if, on some level, I knew Slim wouldn't be with us in physical form for as long as I would wish; I had started collecting documents and recordings of his talks and workshops. This helped enormously in creating this book. As much as was possible, Slim's exact words were cited throughout the book and are **_italicized_** for easy identification. Where it was necessary to improve readability or understanding, careful and minimalistic editing was done.

This book is a reference guide for those of you who have Light-Life Tools, providing detailed information on their many applications and uses. For those unfamiliar with the tools, it is an inspiring read offering ideas for approaches to improve health and the environment. Perhaps your intention is to reduce air pollution, or the effects of electromagnetic fields, or farm with little or no pesticides, or energize food, water, and yourself. The tools can help you attain those objectives and so much more. Let yourself be inspired as you travel through the pages of *In the Mind of a Master.* You're in for quite a ride!

Katharina Spurling-Kaffl

INTRODUCTION

Teachers come into and fade away from our lives continually, leaving their marks behind like fingerprints on a piece of glass. Often this is done without a true awareness of the impact they had on us. Some teachers tell us what it is that we need to learn. Others go a step beyond and explain why it is we need to learn. The good teacher does all of this, then demonstrates how we can achieve what it is we are looking for. The truly great teacher, the master teacher, is the one who completes those steps by inspiring us - inspiring us to achieve; inspiring us to nurture the seedling of potential as it is waiting to emerge; inspiring us to wake up to the limitless possibilities that lay dormant below the surface; inspiring us to mold our learning so that it fits us as an individual rather than trying to create an exact copy of the message we have been presented; inspiring us to reach deep inside, to find that heartfelt song so unique to us that only we can share it with another. One of those master teachers who touched so many lives was Slim Spurling.

My husband Scott and I had the good fortune to have met Slim and attend a few of his workshops relating to geobiology and earth energies between the years 2006-2007. Slim, an unassuming man, taught with a down-home style authenticity that stirred those he connected with to further explore and engage in the healing work he was encouraging. Using his compellingly simple, yet powerfully effective techniques and technology, the average person has the potential to achieve amazing results in environmental and personal self-care.

The intent of this book is to continue to pass along the teachings Slim Spurling selflessly shared with the world. Since he is no longer here in physical form, this will be accomplished by compiling the work Slim presented through the years into a resource that will be a valuable asset for those wishing to learn about Light-Life Technology, as well as for anyone already utilizing this amazing science.

Slim's wife, Katharina Spurling-Kaffl, has generously granted me access to Slim's personal writings, correspondences, workshops, and interviews, both written and taped. This allows the material to come through in Slim's voice as it was actually presented, in most instances. There are a few exceptions. At times, I have edited down Slim's words to allow for a better flow in reading. Also, there are instances when an explanation is needed but I was unable to find any primary source from Slim recorded on that topic. Those gaps have been filled from secondary sources, including Katharina Spurling-Kaffl, other research associates, or myself. As a reminder, you will find the paragraphs with Slim's words *italicized* for easy identification.

Katharina has provided me with field reports sent to Slim and her about the tools. As a teacher myself, it is always my objective to excite the student to see the possibilities and opportunities available through learning. As you read what Slim is telling us, you will learn about the many tools and applications. And, as you hear the remarkable experiences others have shared, you too will be curious to learn more through personal exploration in relation to Slim's discoveries and techniques.

To lay the foundation, basic knowledge about some of the factors influencing personal health and wellness will be introduced. This will be followed with the main portion of the book devoted to the presentation of the tools and their extensive applications. The book also includes valuable field reports provided by research associates from around the world who have shared their individual experiences using the tools. It is my hope you will be inspired to explore them yourself and come up with your own creative applications to help yourself, family, friends, and the greater community at large.

My Introduction to the Tools

My husband Scott and I rented a booth at a local health fair in Pennsylvania to promote our holistic center, Seeds for Change Wellness. Unknown to us at the time, several other similar events were being held in the area as well and therefore attendance was light. Becoming bored, Scott began to visit the other vendors, curious as to what they were endorsing. Each time he would come back excited about some new item he saw. On the second day after his walk around, he came back with a ½ Sacred Cubit Plain Jane Ring. Exasperated with him, I asked, "WHAT did you buy now??" He said it was a healing ring. In his opinion, no one would sit there for two days trying to sell a small ring if it didn't do anything. He put it in his pocket and promptly forgot about it. The ½ Cubit Ring sat on his dresser at home for weeks unnoticed.

Then one evening as Scott was getting ready to leave to play ice hockey, he became aware of a large swollen area over his groin, a possible hernia - not what he wanted to be facing! Dowsing[1] to see if he should play that night, he was surprised to get an OK, so he went. Once home, he remembered the ring sitting on his dresser and the potential it had for accelerating healing. He also recalled the numerous testimonials he had read with complete skepticism. So he went to bed with the ring over his groin to test its healing ability. Knowing he had to make an appointment with the doctor to check if indeed he had a hernia, Scott added an intention that whatever this was, it would heal without needing surgery. When he awoke the next morning, he was startled by the reduction in the size of the swelling. If anything, he thought, after an evening of playing hockey, it should have been worse not better. He immediately woke me up to tell me the news. In my early morning fog, I said, "That's nice" and promptly rolled over and fell back asleep.

Each evening thereafter, Scott continued to follow the same routine using the ring, placing it over the affected area, while stating the personal intention that he did not want to have surgery. In the meantime, he made a few doctor appointments, which were spread over a couple of weeks. The first doctor confirmed he had a hernia, as did the second. His recommendation was to see the workers' compensation doctor, who then also confirmed the diagnosis. Four weeks later, after sleeping with the ring over the swollen area, Scott had an appointment to see a surgeon to schedule the hernia operation. The surgeon did a scan of the area and said, "You don't have a problem. How did they even detect this? There's the tiniest little tear. See me if it ever becomes a problem." After that prognosis, Scott returned to skating and never had an issue with it again.

After his personal experience with the ½ Sacred Cubit Ring, Scott was a believer in this technology. He delved into reading the book *Slim*

---

1 Dowsing is a technique that allows us to gather information not directly available to our conscious mind

Spurling's Universe by Cal Garrison, as well as researching and contacting individuals to learn more about Light-Life Technology. I, on the other hand, was not so convinced. Yes, he did avoid surgery, but really now, how could a simple round circle of twisted copper that did not plug into anything, accomplish that? The skeptic inside had burning questions. My decision: if Scott wanted to continue his explorations of this subject, fine, but I wasn't interested in going along for the ride. At least that is what I initially thought.

Sometimes one needs an epiphany to provide the necessary fuel for change. I am almost embarrassed to say that is exactly what happened in my case. Every now and again I get a reoccurring ache in my left foot. There is no explanation medical doctors can find as to why this develops. When I have what I call an "episode," I am able to provide some form of holistic self-care that allows me to function with minimal distress. Then one "episode" occurred to which my typical treatments did not respond. Being in extreme pain, I was laid up on the sofa. This was more intense than any other time, each day building upon the previous one, with the pain getting worse, until walking on it proved too much. I had run through my standard variety of remedies: Reiki, acupressure, cold pressed castor oil packs, anti-inflammatory supplements, and my LED device for reducing pain - all with no relief. Then at one point, Scott walked into the room and, noticing how badly I was feeling, took the ½ Sacred Cubit Ring out of his pocket. He slipped it over the troubled foot. Too weak to resist, I let it sit there. The most amazing thing happened - within less than one minute, the pain subsided. I sat straight up and said to him, "OK, now you have my attention!" This was probably the single most dramatic shift I had ever experienced in my life, going from a state of intense pain to a state of complete relief. I waited for the pain to return. I wiggled my foot, walked on it, and put my shoe on, with each action expecting to greet the arrival of the pain once again. When my foot remained pain-free, an intuitive leap of understanding took hold. Thus, I joined my husband on the journey of learning, using, and sharing information about the tools. My hope is, whether believer or skeptic, through the sharing of testimonials like ours and others, along with an understanding of the uses of the tools, you will become interested enough to explore more about this technology that holds so much potential.

Susan Anderson

Part I
Laying the Foundation

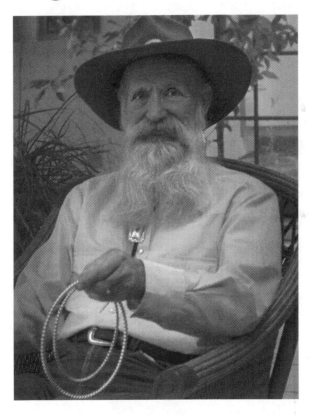

Slim Spurling
1938—2007

NOTES:

CHAPTER 1
Meet the Master ~
An Autobiography of Slim Spurling

I'm Slim Spurling, the discoverer and inventor of a couple processes which we're gonna discuss today. To give you a little bit of background on myself, I was born 1938 in South Dakota near Aberdeen. My first home there was in Bison. My folks were involved in agriculture and my dad was a county agent. Our house was just a little tarpaper shack out there on the dry flats in Bison, South Dakota.

We moved around a lot during the early years, went from Bison to Elgin, Illinois. Dad had a job with the Milwaukee Railroad as an agricultural agent; and when World War II came along, we went from army camp to army camp and spent some time in central South Dakota. I got to know all the plants in the area, and became a self-taught herbalist.

After World War II, my family moved to a small ranch near Morrison, Colorado. Prior to college, I served as a Petty Officer Third Class in the Navy Air Reserve. During that time, I had a chance meeting with the navy commander at the base barbershop. I guess my reserve record and grades impressed my commander, because he wrote a letter exempting me from monthly reserve duties. This conversation turned out to be a significant episode in my life. The next month, while flying to Olathe, Kansas, all the reservists were killed when the flight went down in a storm. Incredibly, this tragic event occurred again the next month as a second flight went down. I was grief-stricken by the loss of my friends, and awed that for some reason, my life had been spared. For the first time, I had the realization that my destiny and purpose for being were guided by forces much larger than I could imagine.

I didn't see myself making a career of the military, and after my enlistment was up, I entered college. Thought that would be a natural way to pursue my interest in the outdoors. I obtained a Bachelor of Science degree at Colorado State University, majoring in forestry and botany, and with a minor in mycology and biochemistry. I took post-graduate seminar courses in chemistry, as well.

As time went on, I became disenchanted with academics. The interest there was to find a chemical substance in the fungus world that could be grown like penicillin and produced very cheaply so that it could be put in as an unregistered and unlabeled ingredient in many different foodstuffs. The purpose of this compound, specifically, according to the details outlined in the protocols of the master's degree program, was to control the population. This was a substance that would lower the threshold of suggestibility and would perhaps have a side effect of producing a mild euphoria.

Now these effects are probably not too alarming, until one considers the social and economic and, perhaps, political considerations for the control of the population. The control of the population was exactly the design parameter of this master's degree program. Well, to make a long story short, it took me three days to locate in the literature that substance, the fungus that produced it, to grow a culture, to ingest a small amount and test it, find out that indeed the effect desired was already known in the literature, but unknown to the designers of this master's program.

Needless to say, I had some ethical and moral considerations there, and I declined to accept the program. In all honesty, I was extremely disgusted and angry to the point of near explosion, so I walked out of Colorado State University a very disillusioned and angry young man. Spent the next twenty years teaching myself the art of blacksmithing, acquired a small shop for a few hundred dollars, and began learning the ancient art of metalworking.

As it turned out, it was a wonderful exercise in alchemy - the ability to deal with four elements in their various forms and qualities - earth, air, fire, and water. So unbeknownst to me at that time, and not even in my consideration, I began to work with these elements and create useful and artistic pieces of metal. After ten years of working solo in my shop and having built it up to a fairly professional level, I opened a school and began to teach the art.

During the time of about five years that the school was open, I had about five helpers toward the end and we had a very large school. It was the largest blacksmith shop in the United States at that time, in the early to mid-70s. I closed the shop down in 1980 and took a job on a ranch. When that proved unsatisfactory, I moved down to Denver and was very much a fish out of water. Having been raised in the country and lived my life there, I found the city life to be a bit disconcerting. I didn't know what to do with myself. I had no job history, no marketable skill in the Denver job market, and about that time I began getting into the metaphysical side of things.

During my years in Denver - I lived there about seven years - I started a little handyman business. Pretty soon I had more work than I could do alone, so I called my old friend Bill Reid and asked him if he needed work or could help. He came over one morning, and we began working together. He was an old friend from many, many years back, and also a physical scientist with a very left-brain approach to physics and chemistry and that type a thing, but still interested in helping me. We began to research the intricacies of alchemy.

I found out that Bill had a tremendous interest in science and some of the more far out, or what we might call fringe science, esoteric things like Nikola Tesla and Wilhelm Reich and scientists that are not mainstream but who had made discoveries which they became famous for. I mentioned Wilhelm Reich data, of which I had read some back in the early 1960s and had built a couple of cloud busters myself. Used them, found them effective, and then found that you didn't need a cloud buster to do the same job. You could do it by throwing energy out through a hand, or just envisioning the energy going out.

Between 1981 and 1989 I did a lot of practice in that area, much to the astonishment of some of the local weathermen, as well as myself. I was riding a tractor one morning up in northern Colorado doing some ranch work. The wind began to blow out of the Laramie area. I noticed kind of a gray, fuzzy, sky. It was not a cloud-bank, but coming in with that wind from Laramie was this blackish stuff floating in the air. I didn't need the wind to come up and blow my cornstalks off to the next county, so I began throwing energy at it. I did that every time I'd head north on the tractor, and I did probably eight or ten rounds of the field and then forgot about it. At the time I noticed the wind starting, I was listening to the KOA weather reports, the farm reports. The announcer was saying, "Well, boys, you've gotta get your baby calves in and make sure you've got plenty of hay in the barn and everything in out of the pastures. We're gonna have a winter storm that is gonna be as bad as any storm we've ever seen. Huge storm coming out of Laramie." Okay, that must be the wind I'm seeing and the gray stuff and I wonder if the gray stuff is associated with it. I didn't know what it was at the time. So the morning passes and the noon farm report came on and the same announcer comes on the radio and he says, "Boys, you're not gonna believe this. That storm vanished. It's gone." And they couldn't explain it. I'm sitting there on my tractor scratching my head, saying, "Wow. This stuff really works, whatever 'it' is."

I knew the feeling. I knew the flow of the energy and the ability to do this, so I spent a year and half playing with cloud patterns and weather, tornadoes, nasty looking thunderstorms, and that kind of thing, but I couldn't teach anybody to do it. They'd look at me like I was totally out of my tree and, matter of fact, the boss told me not to even talk about it. The neighbors were beginning to talk. If you have all the rain you need to raise hay, what else do you need to be concerned about!

So Bill and I began to experiment in the evenings, doing alchemical work. Bill had a lifetime interest in alchemy. He was a mining engineer and metallurgist, having had his own precious metal refinery at one time. Since I'd been out of the science world and the academic world for many, many years, I had to kind of play catch up. I began by listening to Bill. He was talking about "field" this and "field" that and different kinds of energies. I was really in the dark. I didn't have a clue.

Bill and I went to a psychotronics conference. I felt totally like a fish out of water seeing guys like Tom Bearden. I can't remember all their names now, but there were grand old folks in psychotronics and subtle energy work and esoteric things that I couldn't even pronounce. But I made a vow that day as I walked in that I would understand it at some point. That I'd come along and I'd study and I'd try and figure this stuff out.

In the middle of that program, Ralph Blum walked in with his freshly published rune book. Some of you may have seen the runes and worked with them a little bit. He set up his little card table and a folding chair, and set out a couple dozen books. I finally got curious enough and got enough gumption up to walk up and start talking to him. He said, "Here, try it." He had a purple sack of stuff and you reach in and pull out the runes. And I guess it's been ever since then we've been on that path of the Spiritual Warrior. Drawing that rune to begin with kinda backed me up a little bit and really set me back on my heels 'cause I didn't know the full implications at the time.

Bill and I continued to experiment down in the basement with scraps of materials and various kinds of junk we'd picked up in dumpsters and back alleys. We developed this thing called a caduceus coil based on this reading we had done. That led us into a study of subtle energies.

At that time, I was married to a woman named Diane who was probably one of the most gifted clairvoyants I've ever known. She had a library full of metaphysical books that she'd never read. She didn't need them. She just looked, saw it. She tutored me for seven years and brought me a little more up to speed on what metaphysics is and how it works. She was able to see the energies, see them in color and detect the extremely subtle changes in the energy fields or the beams that were projected from these caduceus coils.

So we began to correlate different types of coils, different tunings, and with her gift of being able to see the colors, we knew that a certain color would give a certain effect.

Ultimately, Diane and I parted company, so I had quiet alone time to get in and define all the terms and begin to study and practice and see if all this stuff really worked. So, between 1981 when we married and 1989/90, I was in that mode of learning a new language, a new way of understanding things. I was beginning to see the reality of, as our American Indian people say, the real world - finding out what prayer is, how it works, and that everything I've said or done or thought was a form of prayer – and I made some major changes in my life.

Bill and I researched in that area for about five years, from 1985-1990, and during this time we also began doing the work with geopathic zones. Initially, we didn't have a good language or definition, but as time went on, learned about the Hartmann Grid, geopathic zones being a distinct variety of these negative energies, and different than the Hartmann Grid.

Well, about 1991 I got into a state of bad health myself. I nearly died, but by using the newly discovered energy form, which contained a ring embedded, the condition passed very rapidly. Basically, it saved my life. From that point on, we researched many, many different areas. We developed a tremendous broad range of understanding and almost an unlimited range of application of these tools.

More biographical information on Slim Spurling ...

Slim began practicing the ancient art of dowsing in 1970. In the mid 1980's, Slim and his partner Bill Reid developed geobiology for stress reduction, which many believe to be one of the powerful approaches for recovery and growth of physical and spiritual well-being. Their simple and inexpensive methodology gives individuals the tools to improve their lives and the lives of others by neutralizing negative earth energies in their living and working environment. Slim was an internationally recognized expert in the art and was known for conducting seminars in the U.S., Canada, Europe, South America, and South Africa.

Slim co-founded the Geobiology Research Association in 1993, a network of student-associates who practiced the art of dowsing for diverting geopathic stress to alleviate various physical, mental, or emotional symptoms for members of households or business enterprises. Field reports gathered for over 18 years from practitioners form a body of evidence for the reality of geopathic stress and the fact that it can be eliminated.

Slim developed a keen interest in metaphysics that was inspired and guided by two near-deaths and an out-of-body experience. Slim's life was about seeking knowledge and truth to achieve healing for the planet through the use of tools and healing methods. His heart-felt desire was to help heal our planet and everyone and everything living on it.

In 1991, Slim invented a device now known as the Light-Life™ Ring. Further inventions based on this technology include the Acu-Vac Coil, Feedback Loop, Harmonizer, Nose Mask, Head Mask, Acupressure Tool, Seed of Life, and Lotus Pendant. These tools, which are room temperature superconductors, produce subtle energy effects in areas as diverse as pain relief, enhanced healing ability of the body in injury or illness, improved water quality, air pollution abatement, certain types of insect control, and increased plant growth.

Slim met Katharina Kaffl in the fall of 1997 at his first workshop near Munich, Germany. In 2001, they were married. To Slim's intuitive genius, Katharina brought her extensive professional experience in business, finance, and practice as a healer to their union. Before long, she also became a partner in his creative world of Light-Life Technologies. Katharina managed the business in order to free up Slim, allowing him more time to focus on his research work. During their time together, they created several new lines of products with over 80 items. On a higher level, Katharina and Slim's marriage wed their commitment to each other with their dream of bringing harmony and healing to the world and its entire people.

The techniques and technologies for personal and environmental health are now recognized and put into practice by a growing network of associate researchers worldwide who are keenly interested in these issues.

Slim's passing on November 12, 2007, left a gap no one can fill. He was an extraordinary, yet humble man. He was an enlightened being who saw goodness in everyone he met and a teacher who captured his students' hearts with inspirational stories and wisdom.

I am including a message from Tana Blackmore, a good friend of Slim's and Katharina's. She trusted Tana to offer a clear, authentic dispatch from Slim. Slim was always available for people, and when you read his message, you'll know nothing has changed. May you be comforted and reassured by these words from Slim Spurling ....

SLIM'S MESSAGE TO US THROUGH TANA BLACKMORE THE DAY OF HIS MEMORIAL

Hello everyone. Thank you for coming. I'd like to set the record straight. I did plan to come back, but as with all things in life, that changed. Well, I didn't feel complete, but now I do. Oh, I'll still have a hand in things, but I'm happy here – more peaceful, more clarity. I can do more from here. I always thought it would be fun to attend your own funeral – you know – see the truth of it all.

There is a lot of sadness I'd like to bring comfort to. You see, I haven't gone anywhere – I'm now everywhere. To those who invite me, I will have coffee with you in the morning, walk and talk with you throughout your day.

Many of you think I'll be back. I'll 'walk in' or channel through someone. Now this is important. I won't be walking in, I don't need to. And I will be talking through someone. I chose this person because of her integrity, ability to see the truth, and commitment to my work. It is Katharina, my wife. So, I ask that you honor her, assist her, and encourage her to trust. Katharina, don't worry, this is going to be fun.

I will be chatting with many of you, but remember this. I will not give you your answers or tell you what to do. That's your job.

During my life, not everything I told you was true – but I did not know that at the time. From here, I can see that – so I encourage you to listen carefully to yourself and less to what is going on in the world.

I know I led the war on conspiracy. I condemned the establishment and would have loved to kick some butts into hell. That was my way of stirring the pot so to speak – to wake folks up.

I'd like to leave you with this for now. I built harmonizers to bring harmony. We can't wage war and have harmony at the same time – I ask that you really think about that.

I thank you all, every one of you, for you made my life rich. Look in the mirror more often, smile, and remember – you are never alone – THE UNIVERSE IS WITH YOU!

A Second message from Slim

I have been asked two questions:

- "What did he mean, he didn't tell us the truth?"

  This morning he answered with, *I spoke to a lot of people about a lot of things and subjects. From my viewpoint then, I was unable to give you the whole truth. I can see that now. It is important for everyone to make their own choices, to learn to trust themselves. Life is for each of us to decide. There are enough followers. Be a leader ... of your life, at least.*

- "What about talking through others or just Katharina?"

His answer, *I will be talking to many of you, even sending messages. I will assist each of you in many ways ... as long as it does not interfere in what you choose to experience. When it comes to my work, the future of my work, and evaluating what is best to do or have or create ... Katharina and I will let you know.*

As I said, invite me for coffee some time, I'll be there. God bless.

CHAPTER 2
The Need to Heal

No one questions the need for healing in today's world, traversing the landscape from personal dimensions on through to the global stage. Healing is desired on all levels, in all areas. This includes people, animals, and plants, as well as the environment. In addition, when seeking to restore complete balance and harmony, one often needs to address not only the physical but the mental, emotional, and spiritual planes as well. We are multidimensional beings operating at all of these levels simultaneously. Therefore, the need to go beyond the inventory of symptoms is absolutely necessary. Understanding the root cause of the imbalance must be focused on so it does not return.

As a holistic practitioner, I guess you can say I have traveled the typical pathways to discovery. Once bitten by the healing bug, the journey of a thousand miles started. Each step often took me to yet another *got to have* this amazing tool, technique, tip, program, workshop, seminar, or conference. In the ocean of overwhelming choices, one's head can spin with all the directions you find yourself pulled.

As time passed, I started to settle down. Although still astonished by much of what I encounter, my ability to discern is a bit more sophisticated. There have been a few basic realizations made along the way. While not new to me from an intellectual perspective, once understood at the heartfelt level, these realizations helped shape my individual philosophy and attitude toward healing. Now, you may be thinking what has this got to do with the tools? Actually, quite a bit, as I will explain shortly.

My first true realization was, regardless of how amazing a healing tool or technique may be, there is never one magic bullet that will yield guaranteed results all the time, in all circumstances, for all individuals. This is a result of our individuality. The end diagnosis of the health or environmental challenge may be the same for a large group of people, yet the factors leading up to that diagnosis can be very different. The complexity of each situation dictates strategies that will bring about a rebalancing of the whole. My next realization: *all healing is an inside job* that can be greatly assisted in a variety of ways by outside technology and programs. I want to repeat this because it is so important: the power to heal comes from within each individual. Somewhere along the way, many of us have decided or have been programmed to give away our power rather than to take responsibility for the direction and quality of our health and wellness. In regard to environmental healing, it is often much easier to allow others to take the reins of responsibility rather than choosing to become a steward for the earth. Through these simple personal discoveries, my main focus shifted to self-empowerment coupled with a pro-active attitude.

Taking responsibility requires dedication to creating a lifestyle that best enhances one's commitment to individual and environmental health. This step involves finding approaches that compliment personal goals. Slim's Light-Life™ Technology is a method that can easily be incorporated into one's lifestyle. Since the tools have come into the lives of my family and friends, they have been used with amazing success. The experiences we have had in regard to healing have, at times, seemed almost miraculous. Whether in the arena of personal or environmental health, we have discovered using the tools enhances and amplifies the work being done.

The Light-Life Tools were created as a functional art form. What exactly does this mean? Functional art goes beyond display and moves into the realm of purpose. Slim Spurling, a master of earth stewardship, as well as a gifted craftsman, blended his passions to create a technology that would serve both. He worked selflessly to advance the cleansing and clearing of the environment. It was through the development and use of the Light-Life Technology that he and others could participate in a broad spectrum of supportive activities, some of which include: clearing land and air pollution, enhancing water quality, improving agricultural methods, reducing the effects of wireless technology, and supporting alternative health methods, as well as personal self-care. It is important to note that the tools will not do the work for you, but will assist you in achieving your desired outcome. When Wallace Black Elk, a tribal elder of the Lakota Native Americans, was asked how we can heal Mother Earth, he replied, "She can heal herself; we just have to stop making her sick!" (Farmer, 2/97) A great deal of unnecessary illness and suffering can be circumvented using relatively simple preventive or corrective measures.

CHAPTER 3
Geobiology and Earth Energies

Geobiology: The study of the influence of "earth energies" on all forms of life: man, animal, and plant. Normally silent and invisible, these energy fields are felt by many and affect lives in profound ways.

Earth energies occur naturally all over the planet, forming a web-like grid around, through, and above the earth. These earth energies can be both positive and negative, or referred to as beneficial and detrimental, in their impact on those that live and work in or near them. Ancient people knew how to identify areas of positive earth energy, often called Ley Lines, where they built churches, stone circles, and other sacred areas. They also knew how to detect areas where earth energies were harmful (geopathic stress). These harmful areas were often found near, around, and above earthquake faults, fissures, underground streams, natural gases, and underground mineral deposits. Ancient people avoided these areas.

With small, mobile populations and abundant land, it was relatively easy to avoid the negative areas of high geopathic stress. However, over the past 100 years, geopathic stress has grown to the extent that it now wraps almost the entire earth in a negative energy grid. The growth in geopathic stress is thought to be largely due to the electrification of the world. Additionally, other man-made developments such as landfills, gas lines, telephone lines, security systems, etc., have been linked to naturally occurring negative earth energy lines, grids, and fields.

More About Geobiology

In very basic terms, geobiology is the study of unseen or invisible energies that emanate from the earth having an effect on living organisms. Every ancient culture had some tradition that incorporated aspects of geobiology, as Slim has mentioned above. The practice of Feng Shui from China is one example, which focuses on the inter-relationship between human beings and the subtle energies of nature. Keep in mind that geobiology goes well beyond the simplified definition provided above. It is humbling as one begins to investigate this subject in depth, realizing the complexity of the topic and how much is yet to be discovered.

Viewed from the western perspective, geobiology is the art of identifying earth energies found in our environment that may have a direct correlation on such things as health, wellness, relationships, and finances. These can appear as subtle yet powerful energies, capable of having either an invigorating, draining, or neutral effect upon living organisms. Once these lines of energy are located and identified, the information can be useful when making decisions, particularly about placement of objects in the local environment. This may include helping to determine the best location and orientation of new properties, homes, buildings, or outdoor landscaping. Inside, it may be useful in selecting the best placement for one's workspace or sleeping quarters, or other areas where a large amount of time is spent on a consistent basis.

As technology advances, it becomes difficult to avoid being immersed in an energetic soup of electromagnetic and microwave pollution. Research now abounds indicating detrimental effects from long-term exposure. Dr. Robert O. Becker, in his ground-breaking book, *Cross Currents*, has written extensively about many of these studies. He states, "Our ability to generate the entire spectrum of electromagnetic fields is a two-edged sword. With no understanding of the relations of these fields to living organisms, we have produced a global environmental alteration that has profound implications for human health. Now that we have finally become aware of the serious consequences of this mistake, we have the responsibility to take actions to reduce this threat to future generations. At the same time, as we learn more about the subtleties of the relationship between electromagnetic energy and living organisms, we will acquire increased knowledge of how living things function. This knowledge will better enable us to use electromagnetic energy in our social and economic affairs and in our medical care systems. The new paradigm of life energy and medicine has the capacity to produce a better world for our children, if we act wisely and quickly."

As our awareness in the field of geobiology increases, we have a means to detect imbalances so a course of action can be taken to help restore balance and harmony. As part of the process inherent in the work, geobiology becomes a tool bridging the connection between the spirit of Mother Nature and human consciousness. Nature is seen as an active and creative presence. The earth is regarded as a living, conscious organism. Once we fully realize the importance of this relationship, we know any imbalance in our surroundings is reflected back at us, creating an imbalance for all the inhabitants of the earth.

EARTH ENERGIES

As if it were a body with its own metabolism, the "wind" and "water" flow, and circulation of negative earth energies has been studied at great length. Proof is with us here and now that the earth is threaded with magnetic lines - meridian points of acupuncture - and our ancient people knew of these points. These points still retain their vibratory intensity and their powerful influence on people. Called in German "Orte der Kraft" they are defined as locations or sites endowed with an energy, a force, a strength.

EARTH ENERGY LINES DEFINED

Ley Lines are positive lines usually found at locations of sacred sites, churches, stone circles, or beneficial natural phenomena. Except in rare occasions, these lines are relatively far apart, 50 miles or more. It is not necessary to clear them. However you may want to locate gardens, fountains, a favorite chair, sacred objects or a bed over Ley Lines.

Geopathic Stress Lines/Zones include the Hartmann Grid, other geopathic stress either natural or man-made, personal zones, interference zones, and vortexes.

The Hartmann Grid was discovered by and named for a German medical doctor, Ernst Hartmann. It is believed to be a result of the electrification of the world and encompasses the earth in a net-like pattern flowing from south to north and west to east. Some pure areas, sacred sites, or very remote areas have no Hartmann Grid, and some have the grid as close as every one to two feet. There appears to be a neutral area between the lines, but the intersection of the lines is believed to be the most harmful place. The centerline is one inch, the Zone of Influence is between 8 - 12 inches, and the grid can reach heights of up to 600 feet.

Other Geopathic Lines/Zones include both natural lines such as earthquake faults or underground water, and manmade lines such as underground gas, sewer, and quarries. These lines are random in nature, though some may be grid-like and are horizontal, vertical, or diagonal.

Personal Lines/Zones can affect individuals differently. These lines can be similar to music, which grates on one person's nerves and yet is enjoyable to another. Typical lines in the category are health, relationships, and finance. A property may have no personal lines, or as many as five or more personal lines per person. The centerline is one inch, the Zone of Influence is variable, and these lines can reach variable heights.

Interference Lines/Zones affect, in a negative/non-supportive way, the goals a property owner or tenant has for their life or property. Basically these lines get in the way of what a person wants, and thus are specific to the intentions the owners/tenants have set. Examples of these lines are: communication, neighbors, and sale of property. A property may have zero interference lines or several. The centerline is one inch, the Zone of Influence is variable, and these lines can reach variable heights.

Vortexes are swirls of earth energy, often with a tornado-type spin, which usually come up from the earth or go down into the earth. You can see evidence of vortexes by noticing twisted tree trunks next to trees of the same species that stand straight and tall. There are both positive and negative vortexes. Not every property has them. It is only necessary to identify the negative vortexes, which spin counter clockwise.

We have found that all lines can be significantly expanded around a full moon.

MORE ON EARTH ENERGIES

Everything in the universe has energy, and all energy vibrates. All vibrations have three characteristics: frequency, wavelength, and amplitude. Frequency can be defined as the rate of vibration. All electromagnetic waves have their own particular frequency signature or rate. This corresponds to the number of changes in direction they make per second. So a frequency can be measured or converted into cycles per second (CPS) or Hertz (Hz). Wavelength is the measure of the length of the cycle. The electromagnetic wave spectrum is a scale of vibration. Two objects whose electromagnetic fields are the same operate at the same frequency. This is called resonance or harmony. Amplitude refers to the length and width of waves, such as sound waves, as they move or vibrate. An important physical variance exists between different substances related to the density or amplitude of their vibration.

Stated simply, the physical body has a vibrating energy field that interacts with other energy fields. Depending on their relative phase or state of vibration, these waves interact or interfere with each other, meaning they can reinforce or cancel one another. A sympathetic reaction (resonance) occurs when vibrations combine harmoniously. A classic example of this is when one tuning fork vibrates at a particular frequency and then is able to activate into motion another tuning fork of similar frequency without actually coming into physical contact.

Going further, one can examine an aspect of resonance called entrainment. This occurs when two or more oscillating objects lock into a cycle so they are synchronized in their vibrations. This concept was first put forth by the Dutch scientist Christian Huygens in 1665. Working with clocks in close proximity of each other, he found that if he swung their pendulums at different rates they would eventually swing together in unison. It was discovered "when two or more objects produce oscillations in close proximity, the dominant frequency will prevail. Eventually they will entrain together into a unified frequency." (Seaward).

Dissonance is yet another characteristic of vibrational behavior. When two waves vibrating at different frequencies meet, they create chaos, clash, or cancel each other out. Take, for example, two children standing together tossing pebbles into a pond. Depending on the timing and proximity of their tosses, some of the ripples created will combine with one another; others will clash or cancel each other. Those that combine, resonate together; those that cancel each other are discordant. Examples of resonance, entrainment, and dissonance are everywhere. Once we really begin to understand these connections, it is easier for us to understand how the various energy fields that surround the physical body are affected by one another.

The earth and all other living organisms are both transmitters and receivers of energy. As a transmitter, energies are constantly broadcasted. As a receiver of earth energies, most human bodies, for example, are only capable of physically sensing a small portion of the surrounding vibrations. There are however, exceptions, as some individuals are extremely sensitive to changes in earth energies. Through the normal sensory pathways, visible light and color is seen with the eyes; sound is perceived through the ears. Other energies, such as x-rays, ultraviolet rays, microwaves, and radio waves are only detectable through science and technology. The nature of the exchange of these various energies between the earth and its inhabitants creates patterns of disbursement that have a broad range of effects.

As stated earlier, earth energies create a grid-like covering over the entire earth. Some of the energies included within this grid: underground waterways, Hartmann Lines, Ley Lines, Schumann Resonance, and vortex energy.

Surrounding the earth is a natural magnetic field. This acts as a force field protecting the earth and all of life from solar radiation. Scientists believe this magnetic field emanates from electrical currents coming from the molten liquid core at the earth's center.

As humans, our bodies are naturally attuned to the electromagnetic field. Other species such as whales, birds, and bees are thought to use this magnetic field for their migration routes. Small fluctuations occur regularly throughout the day, but are barely noticed. Most individuals are able to handle the variations, some of which are results of weather conditions or sun activity.

Geopathic stress is not only limited to planetary events. Cyclical sunspot activity, with accompanying solar storms, can also create stressful situations for our planet. A strong solar flare can result from a violent eruption on the surface of the sun, and the resulting radioactive waves might be felt on earth within minutes. Depending on the intensity of these waves, communications and electrical fields could be disrupted. A Coronal Mass Ejection (CME) moves much slower, usually taking up to three days to reach earth, but when these plasma filled particle clouds interact with earth's magnetic fields, they have the capability of producing strong geomagnetic storms. While the global electric power grid and communications are vulnerable to the damage that these storms may produce, researchers are also evaluating whether there is a relationship between earthquakes and solar activity.

CHAPTER 4
Geopathic Stress Zones

A geopathic stress zone is an area which brings about pathological conditions in plants, the human body, or an animal body. Geopathic stress zones tend to have negative or chaotic energy fields. A negative spin that causes a negative effect in the body produces high levels of stress. Where these zones cross a bed or a favorite sitting chair or an area of the home where a person may stand or sit for a long period of time, or in the workplace at a desk, can get very, very uncomfortable. And it is the type of stress that comes on unseen - you can't see it, hear it, smell it, or taste it - unless you are clairvoyant or sensitive. Many of the sensitives in our acquaintance are able to see these fields or zones, and also can hear them. Some of them experience a change in taste or maybe a prickling or uncomfortable feeling somewhere in the body when they experience this resonant pattern, or this disturbed pattern, which is out of resonance or out of sync with their own bio-field.

With our rapid technological advancements today, we are contributing enormously to the amount of geopathic stress in our environment. This occurs as a result of the electromagnetic fields caused by electrical and wireless sources. The short list includes such things as: excessive use of electricity, bleeding wires, appliances, lighting, computers, TV, cell phones, transformers, power lines, generators, and all our wireless gizmos and gadgets.

Depending on the source, these energies can vary in intensity, direction, and form. Some are found in regularly spaced grid patterns, where others may be more random in width and structure. Experts estimate that 5% of the earth is covered by them. As one would think, areas of energy intersections are especially troublesome.

When we analyze the word geopathic stress, *geo* refers to the earth, while *pathic* refers to suffering or disease. In combination with stress, it refers to any type of noxious energies, natural or man-made, that over time may create health challenges for humans, plants, and animals under its influence. In addition, inanimate objects are also subjected to its powerful force. Very few things can avoid being affected.

WHY DO WE CARE ABOUT GEOPATHIC STRESS?

Studies have shown the presence of high levels of radioactivity, infrared radiation, and electromagnetic field strength precisely over water veins, fault zones, and areas of geo-magnetic disturbance as indicators of geopathic stress. Geopathic stress is associated with a high percentage of illness.

Certain health professionals in the U.S.A., Europe, and elsewhere who are aware of the negative effects of geopathic stress zones either through scientific research or intuitively, recommend their patients do not return to the same sleeping/working location after successful treatment for various health problems.

A partial list of the health effects of sleeping, living, or working in a high geopathic stress zone is shown below:

Sleep disorders, tingling, numbness and/or pains in the extremities, chronic fatigue, aching and swollen knees, dizziness, frequent headaches, vision problems, disorientation, memory loss, irritability, stress, swollen abdomen, nausea, open sores unable to heal, allergies, and problems with menstrual cycles. Other health problems directly or indirectly attributed to geopathic stress may include cancer, especially leukemia and brain cancer, neurological disability, and cardiovascular issues.

Certain ailments and disorders seem to be linked to particular types of geopathic stress. For example, hyper functioning disorders such as fatigue, arthritis, cancer, multiple sclerosis, and degenerative conditions can be found above mineral ore deposits or earthquake fault lines. Hypo functioning disorders such as hypertension, apoplexy, "mania" types of psychological disorders, and alcoholism can be found above water veins or caverns. Fatigue, chronic skin complaints, and degenerative conditions can be found in low-level areas of radiations such as granite/underground oil shales and in high-level radiation ores. Geopathic stress zones create energy fields with high positive ions. These positive ions actually have a negative impact on human life and on many animals and plant life. Areas with minimal or no geopathic stress zones produce negative ions, which are generally beneficial for health.

Slim Discusses His Early Experiences

I should probably start with the events that got me on the path of healing myself – on the path of discovery, as it were. These were things I had no precedent for in my experience, and the results were phenomenal, to say the least. My discoveries were beyond anything I might have expected, and I give a lot of credence to some of the metaphysical things I've heard about, or was beginning to hear about, and also which take us back into history, perhaps thousands, or even hundreds of thousands of years.

I'll lay out the first scenario where I used dowsing and the "acupuncture" technique that I'm currently using for diverting the grid energies away from the home or business.

I'm going to try to give you a little bit of an idea of the area. On the west side of Denver are the mountains. As you approach that area, you're always impressed with these Hogback Mountains. They're just this narrow-lipped edge, they come up and run, oh, a mile or two in length, and the creek will come winding down through them. So my old-time home, there since 1946, was right on Bear Creek just east of the mountains. We had a 60-acre property there, and I lived right on Bear Creek. Along the bottom of the Hogbacks ran the county road, running fairly straight along there. There were a couple of natural lakes called the Soda Lakes, which have a rather interesting history. The early pioneers used to boil the water, boil it down pretty dry and recover soda ash for washing clothes and their traveling gear. There was an old Indian campground on both sides of the creek, high stream banks there cut through by the streams. I lived there for about 35 years. I called it home.

In 1980, we suddenly began noticing a number of accidents that would occur right about this particular location on the road. Every car hit exactly the same spot. If you'd driven a stake in there, everyone would hit that stake. I was curious about that. How come all of a sudden we have all these accidents? So I'd been reading a little book by Harvey Howells called "Dowsing for Everyone." Anyway, in this book, he described geopathic zones.

The term he used was zones of noxious energy. So along in the book, one of the stories was about dowsers using different means to block these energy zones and bring about improvements in health or sleeping patterns. One of the stories involved blocking a zone outside of an intersection where there'd been a high number of accidents. So I wondered if these accidents had been caused by geopathic stress.

Well, I went down the road and dowsed for about half a mile. Right at this location, I found a stream crossing that went into the small lake, and I knew there was a little spring up on the hillside, kind of a marshy area. I suspected that there might be a crack or a fissure deep in the earth and that the stream pretty much followed that water course. At that point, I took a couple of rods, once I'd located it, and since I was standing right on the spot where the rods had opened, and I thought well, maybe these will work. Let's see if I can block that energy from crossing the road if that's what's causing the problem. So I knelt down and just stuck them into the ground and shoved the handles down just a couple feet off the road in the grass. So we'd gone from the historical rate of one or two accidents a year, to steadily climbing to maybe one every two or three months. If we graph this and show the historical trend, we'd see a curve of one or two a year, finally up to one or two a month in later times, as traffic increased and they'd paved the road and so on and so on. And in 1979, this curve went suddenly like this, up to 20 a day. It was carnage. Well, that coincided with the grand alignment with the planets in May of 1980. So to make a long story short, this accident rate from the time I blocked this, as far as I know to the present time, went straight down to zero. We had a spike, then a zero, and it didn't return to its historical normal as long as I was in that area. And as I drove past that area 15 years later, I didn't see any evidence of accidents in that particular area. 'Course it's a four-lane highway now. But you know, this to me was unbelievable. I had no precedent, total left-brain at the time, I'm saying, Okay - we have a series of accidents that happen every day. The helicopters and sirens are overhead. This is not possible. So, as I left my old home ground, a lot of my paradigm shifted.

GEOPATHIC STRESS AND ILLNESS

Geopathic stress seems to depress the immune system when a living organism finds itself sitting, working, or sleeping in an area that is geopathically stressed for several hours at a time, on a continual basis. For example, if there is a line of geopathic stress flowing through your bedroom at the location of your bed, in particular where you are sleeping, you can assume you are not sleeping in a safe place. Chances are high you are not sleeping well at all. Even more likely, the exact position where the line of geopathic stress crosses your body may be the exact location where you are experiencing health problems.

Every person is different; some people are more sensitive and easily affected, others may seem to remain totally unaffected, and still others fall somewhere in between the two extremes. When someone is ill and has tried a number of different approaches to healing without success, then it may be time to examine the concept of geopathic stress as a contributing factor. Those who seem to heal, and then have a reoccurrence, also should take time to examine this as a possibility.

Headaches, tumors, and cancers, by the way, are a disease of location. Cancer always occurs in the location where two of these zones cross in a person's bed. If it's in the upper body, it'll be in the throat and the tissue in the lungs. You'll see cancers on the legs and feet anywhere in the world, but they'll always be on those crosses. The Hartmann brothers, one a doctor and the other an engineer, from Germany did a study on this back in the 1940s, I think. They documented 5,000 cases. There was a 98% correlation with the cross in the geopathic stress with the occurrence of cancer. Generation after generation of succeeding family owners in homes where two zones crossed had cancer. It's due to the particular energy in that house and the oddity that everybody parks their bed in exactly the same place in the room, and the guy sleeping on that side of the bed gets cancer and the one on the other side doesn't. And that's the simple reason. And the reason is, it's a one-inch band of energy that crosses the bed. Where two of those intersect and cross, that's where you'll have cancer. It brings on all of the other degenerative diseases, and we've seen everything from MS, to cancer, to chronic fatigue syndrome all resolved, all going away after doing geopathic stress work, knocking out/ neutralizing these zones. So I can comfortably say that geopathic stress is at the root at every known ailment, whether it's physical, emotional, mental, or spiritual.

In our research, the first time out that we did an experiment, we were very fortunate. We were called to a lady's home to do some house repairs. I'd worked for her previously and found her to be quite a delightful woman - young, blonde, early thirties, obviously fairly well-to-do, and living in a nice district with a very nice home. When I'd been there before, she treated me wonderfully well, stopped for coffee, and fixed some fruit and cake, not the usual thing when you're raking leaves and hauling trash and trimming trees.

We got to the door on this second call, and she met us and her face was kind of pinched in and she didn't look like the same person I remembered. She didn't have the same aura about her, the same attitude, and she was a bit crabby. Bill says, "I don't want to work for her. Let's get out of here." I said, "Hey wait a minute. That's not the same person that I know. Let's find out more about this."

As time went on, we found out that she had gotten a migraine headache the day she moved in the house, and she'd had it continuously for three years. She'd traveled over half the planet and spent in excess of $40,000 searching for a specialist who could help get rid of her headache. And nobody had. We thought, well let's ground her gutters, make sure the electricity is flowing in the right direction through the house, and do a couple other things. We found that her furnace was out of adjustment and was producing a little carbon monoxide. We made a slight change for her over a period of a couple of weeks.

Then one day we came by the house and decided to dowse for negative energy. We'd heard about it, but never experienced it or done any dowsing for that particular item. Well, about every ten feet going along the side of her house we'd find this place where the dowsing rods would open and there'd be a distinct feeling there. It didn't feel good. So we used a simple technique to remove the negative energy from her home. Since she wasn't home that day, we were unable to talk to her. We went back three days later and spoke with her, and she reported that she had a complete absence of a headache on that particular day.

I said, "Well, Bill and I came by and we stopped and moved the geopathic zones we found there. That happened about 3 o'clock in the afternoon." She said, "Well I got home at four and my house was crystal clear!" This dark, heavy energy had completely vanished and she was actually able to see the difference. She said, "I woke up the next morning totally without pain for the first time in three years." So that was where we started and how the first incident of our dowsing for geopathic stress occurred.

Noxious Energies and Zones of Disturbance

Noxious energies and zones of disturbance are terms that come to mind when describing geopathic stress. Here, we are referring to any distorted earth energy that, when exposed for prolonged periods of time, can create havoc on the immune systems of most living organisms, although some organisms thrive in these zones.

Geopathic stress is believed to be caused by the otherwise natural healing vibrations of the earth being affected when encountering subterranean running water, faults, and certain mineral deposits. Also amplifying these noxious radiations are loose energies from man's overuse of electricity and wireless technologies in the form of bleeding wires, transformers, and cell phones. These energies are believed to be attracted to subterranean water forming three dimensional rivers of concentrated radiations. Experts believe that these radiations are 300-400 times more intense than they were 100 years ago, mainly due to man's activities.

Ranchers have long observed animals, such as sheep and oxen, as they were herded across the land. They instinctively circumvented geopathic stress, and this information was used in building site selection. Animals such as horses, dogs, pigs, mice, goats, chickens, swallows, and fish all are known geopathic stress avoiders. Although dogs typically avoid geopathic stress, I know of two cases where the dog actually frequented geopathic stress locations in the home, probably to protect the family. Both dogs developed illnesses, including cancerous growths, which resulted in premature death. Geopathically stressed cows tend to lose their natural sheen, have more mastitis, and lower milk yield. Pigs react to geopathic stress by developing black spots. Piglets become restless, wean poorly, and have a higher death rate.

Oddly enough, there are geopathic stress seekers which will thrive in certain radiations. They include: ants, bees, wasps, beetles, and termites. Ant nests are often located over the junction of underground streams. Bees will typically produce more honey in a hive over geopathic stress. Molds, mildews, bacteria, viruses, cats, owls, and snakes are all attracted to geopathic stress (Anderson).

SOME OF THE SIGNS AND SYMPTOMS OF GEOPATHIC STRESS

One of the symptoms of geopathic stress after a very long term is adrenal exhaustion. So if any of you are practitioners and your clients are exhibiting signs of adrenal exhaustion, be sure you have a practitioner who can go out in the field and do the geopathic work for them. Recommend that. Another symptom you'll find is the roller coaster effect. They'll come in right here at the bottom of the pit and your practice brings them up to a high, and then when they leave and go back home, they're back down in the pit again in about a week. Knock out the geopathic stress, and they'll come back here and they'll plateau and go on at a newer, higher level.

Geopathic stress leaves its calling card for all to see. Once you are familiar with some of the warning indicators, an assessment can be fairly simple to determine if your home or business is affected. Good dowsing and observation skills can also help with this process. Below is a list of signs and symptoms commonly associated with geopathic stress.

Environmental Clues: Here are some environmental clues that could indicate geopathic stress may be present at your property site: problems with mold in the house; moss growing on the roof, walls, or lawn; problems with termites, ants, wasps, or bees; cracks in walls, driveways, paving stones, curbs, and roads; reoccurring mechanical and electrical breakdowns; areas with high rates of accidents; presence of trees with cancer, gaps in hedges, rows or shrubs, infertile fruit trees, strangely twisted trees, areas where nothing will grow, or where growth is stunted or mutated; areas susceptible to lightning strikes.

Personal/Health Related Clues: Other observations and questions to ask include: has someone in the home had a serious health challenge or illness which does not heal despite good treatment; does the house seem to drain your energy; do you feel better when you are away from the home, then become weak, energetically depleted or sick once returning to the house; were you in good health and then became ill shortly after moving into the home; do you live in a house which has never "felt right," with some areas so uncomfortable you avoid them; do you wake up in the morning feeling exhausted despite having a full night's sleep; do you suffer from insomnia; do you have close neighbors who may be in poor health; were the previous owners of the home ill?

My husband and I are dowsers who have been doing energy clearing work for the past few years on properties. We have encountered a variety of interesting cases. In most situations, the homeowners were experiencing some level of personal difficulties. Examples include insomnia, asthma, high concentrations of EMFs, cancers, uncomfortable energy within the home, difficulties with interpersonal relationships among family members, repeated mechanical and electrical breakdowns, inability to sell a home, lack of abundance, and multiple chemical sensitivities. Once a property is assessed through dowsing, the location where geopathic stress is found is then remediated using the best selected technique for that particular situation. Often within an hour or two, the energy in the home shifts, and the homeowners recognize the improvement.

Robert Becker, M.D., author of the *Body Electric and Cross Currents* and one of the most respected research scientists in this area, stated, "We now live in a sea of electromagnetic radiation that we cannot sense and that never before existed on this earth. New evidence suggests that this massive amount of radiation may be producing stress, disease, and other harmful effects all over the world by interfering with the most basic levels of brain function." *(How Electromagnetic Radiation Becomes Your Invisible Killer).*

With increasing amounts of distorted earth energies appearing on the local and global scene, it is time to get the word out. People need to be aware of the existence of this phenomenon and learn how to remediate its affects so the pain and suffering associated with it can be reduced. Slim Spurling's Light-Life™ Tools and Technology offer a means to work with rebalancing our environment in a non-intrusive way without creating an additional burden on the earth.

RESULTS OF REMOVING GEOPATHIC STRESS

In removing geopathic stress from a home or business, we found the usual thing that happens is that people have more energy. Initially they may feel so tired that they just crash for twenty-four or forty-eight hours. As the stress is relieved, they just kinda let their breath out and report that they really need to go sleep and just relax. The reason for that is that geopathic stress affects the level of adrenal flow from the kidneys, and you have a constant irritation, constant pressure, and a constant adrenaline rush that you're not even quite aware of.

CHAPTER 4

DRAVET SYNDROME AND THE RINGS

"My friend, Tammy, has a six-year old daughter with Dravet Syndrome, which is a seizure disorder. She can have up to 20 seizures a day. When I talked to Katharina Spurling about this little girl and her situation, Katharina suggested that geopathic stress might be the source of the problem because she suffered more seizures at home than any other place. She gave me the Advanced Dowsing Set. I placed four sets of three rings overlapping in each corner of Destiny's bedroom over two weeks ago. These sets were comprised of four ½ Sacred Cubit Plain Jane Rings, four 1 Sacred Cubit Plain Jane Rings, and four 1 Lost Cubit Plain Jane Rings. Additionally, I placed a silver plated Sacred Cubit Environmental Harmonizer in their family room. Since that time, Destiny has not had one seizure in her home." *A.H., CO*

SLIM SPURLING ANSWERS QUESTIONS ABOUT GEOPATHIC STRESS

QUESTION: I have kidney problems related to varicose veins. It sounds like I must have a Hartmann Line crossing some place in my area. What are your thoughts?

SLIM: *Yeah, the geopathic zone lowers the resistance and interferes with the immune system so that we pick up chronic conditions such as viruses, bacteria, fungus, and other parasites. I lump parasites into those specific classes - the whole range of organisms that commonly inhabit our bodies and finally take over, and down we go.*

I'm going to bring in here a thought that I had this morning. In scripture, you remember somewhere in there, someone may know exactly where it is - old Lucifer's talking and he says, "I will cast a net upon the whole earth." It could be that the Hartmann Grid and the geopathic zones are that net, because they are defined as chaos zones and introduce chaos into otherwise orderly and organized systems. Our bodies are basically very orderly and organized systems created, obviously, by the One Being. So, if that be true, we found a way at least to lift a portion of that net so it doesn't bother us.

QUESTION: What are some observations you have made after clearing geopathic stress?

SLIM: *Some of the interesting things we observed after the geopathic stress lines are neutralized is bird life seems to increase in the area. Even in small yards, it seems like the backyard is full of birds. They love to come in and be in that space, and other creatures as well. Sometimes squirrels, raccoons, and other animals will come in to the area. Ants, on the other hand, tend to disappear after you've neutralized the geopathic stress. We've seen quite a number of cases. Probably the best recommendation I had on that, and one of the nicest reports, came from the president of a major oil company in Dallas. We had the opportunity to clear a home for him. The purpose was to relieve some stresses that he was undergoing. That was resolved, and we heard when the exterminator came to check the house in the spring, he couldn't find any cockroaches or ants. He said, "Gee, I'm sorry, but I can't charge you for my services."*

QUESTION: Can geopathic stress affect inanimate objects in a room?

SLIM: *Of interest to you would be the fact that my partner Bill Reid went to a jazz concert one night and he quickly dowsed the concert hall. He got acquainted with the piano player and the guy says, "I can't make this thing work right. This piano isn't right for some reason." He was also a piano tuner, so he got in there and he tuned on it awhile. Couldn't make the thing sound just the way he wanted it. So Bill says, "Wait a minute. Let's check something." So he got his dowsing rods and checked, and there was a geopathic zone going right across the piano. So, he took an omega coil and taped it to the wall. He checked a few more, especially where the group would have been working. The musicians normally played for an hour at a sitting. That evening, they played for three and a half hours without a break, felt wonderful, and said it was the best performance they had ever given as a group. And, incidentally, the piano sounded the best that it could possibly sound.*

So these geopathic zones introduce a dissonance, if you will, into the environment, and they can actually affect physical things like steel piano strings and guitar strings, as well as the quality of the voice coming through a microphone. But just be aware that a voice, when projected through a ring, makes quite a difference in the way it would sound to you out there in the back room.

QUESTION: What happens when you block geopathic zones or lines? Where does the energy go?

CHAPTER 4

SLIM: *It's very, very simple. It's just like you throw a rock in a river. The water goes over the rock. The clairvoyants see the energies going like this. Why it works that way, I don't know. All I know is that it does work, so I'll leave that to the bean counters and the quantum physicists to figure out. We're only interested in the practical aspects of it to know how to help ourselves, our families, and our friends.*

We started this, oh gosh, in '85. Bill Reid and I were partnered up in a little handyman business. I mentioned the story about the gal who had the chronic migraine and she was cured of that malady. We've looked back on that over the past twelve, thirteen years, and we still marvel at the simplicity of what we did and how well it worked for her.

Then we went on and began doing the same service for others we ran into in our business, and we found that all sorts of physical maladies could be alleviated, if not completely removed. I think our next case was an area where a lot of men were having heart attacks. Matter of fact, one gentleman actually died during the time we were working in that area. We didn't have the opportunity to do his home, although I knew him and he showed no signs of heart problems. He was a happy, healthy guy. And, boom, all of a sudden he went down with a heart attack. But we did do several other homes in the neighborhood. The gentlemen in question all reported relief from this contraction they were having and the heart problems they'd suffered for years.

And I personally experienced a very local phenomenon. I slept in the bed of a person who'd died of a heart attack, and when I woke up in the morning, my heart was in spasm. I was in a lot of pain, and experiencing a lot of difficulty, so the next night I just changed ends in the bed. I slept the other way and I didn't have the same symptoms. The symptoms relieved later in the day. I found my dowsing spot under where my heart was positioned, and discovered there was a crossing. So, it's very real to me. Those of you who may have other difficulties or symptoms or even a generalized kind of malaise, or you just don't feel good - you take the geopathic stress out. Your overall health and well-being will improve. We have a lot of recent cases in California where that's proved to be true. My friend Dorothy's neighbor was down with, I don't know, some cancer, or just didn't feel good, or a combination of things. She'd been bedridden, as a matter of fact, and after they did the geopathic zones, she was up and awake, and bright and healthy, and really made a dramatic recovery in a few weeks. So this was the kind of thing that can happen. It won't happen in every case. But probably 90 - 95%, maybe 98%, will get relief.

CHAPTER 5
Dowsing ~ What Is It?

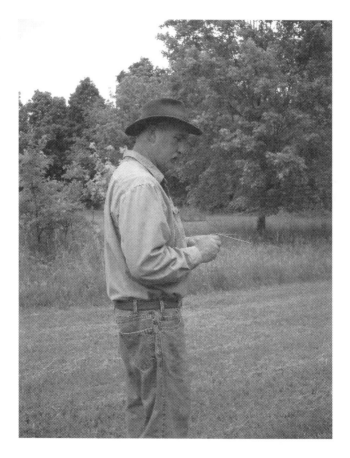

"There's no magic to it.
I just pay attention and experiment."

Slim Spurling

REDISCOVERING DOWSING

All things, whether living or inert, give off energetic radiation. Our own senses can feel and measure these energies. One method of communication used to translate these energies between the conscious and subconscious mind is a technique called dowsing.

In today's society, dowsing is slowly being rediscovered as a useful tool, as we reawaken to our innate abilities. The American Society of Dowsers, which started with a small group of interested individuals in 1961, has grown today to over 3000 members. A quick search of the Internet can lead one to a vast collection of workshops, conferences, organizations, and reference materials on this topic. As the consciousness of the planet shifts into a new paradigm, techniques such as dowsing will be viewed in a different light. Previously scoffed at by modern day scientists as lacking credibility, skilled dowsers today successfully locate long-lasting sources of water and oil. Their results are stunning and elevate dowsing to a legitimate art. Through fields of study such as quantum physics, science may soon catch up with what is already intuitively known by many. The wheels of change are turning. As we expand our awareness, we accept that there are forces outside of our realm of understanding. They may not be identifiable by traditional scientific terms, but may provide us with better ways of doing things. In the context of this book and the teaching methods employed by Slim Spurling, dowsing is an important skill to be mastered, especially when working with geopathically stressed areas.

Dowsing is a common practice in many cultures, which dates back thousands of years. It is easily learned and is particularly useful in identifying the earth energy lines, both positive and negative, which cause an impact in our homes, communities, and workspaces. It is fairly common in the U.S. culture to use a dowser to locate water or other underground lines, though less common to use it to identify and divert negative energy lines. Dowsing is an excellent tool for locating and diverting negative earth energies.

Dowsing is an art, which interfaces the unseen world with our energy body and can be thought of as our intuition communicating with us through dowsing tools. Dowsing is as simple as asking and watching the dowsing instrument for the answer. The key to dowsing is to ask clear questions with a clear intention.

Dowsing is easy to do and easy to learn. Women tend to learn it more quickly and can be better at it than men, but anyone can learn it. Even a child can do it. Almost anything can be used to dowse. Many old-time dowsers dowse with the branches from certain trees, such as willow, apple, or ash, and others use a pendulum. You can also dowse just using your body! As you become more tuned in, you will "feel" the answers. Many people start with a pendulum or "L" rods or even a willow branch. Most people will have a preference, finding it easier to work with one or another. What you use to dowse is less important than having a clear intention. Even if you already know how to dowse with a pendulum, it is helpful to learn dowsing with "L" rods, as they work well in helping identify geopathic stress lines and verifying the direction of the flow of the lines.

Dowsing for natural oil and gas works well when the dowser and a geologist work together. Seismic surveys, accurate for indicating structures, are not always correct when indicating hydrocarbon areas. Dowsing at a site of interest for hydrocarbon bearing areas increases the likelihood of confirming natural oil and gas. One of my students retired in his 40s as a multi-millionaire using the techniques he learned from me and applied them to dowse for oil.

Anyone can practice dowsing without a license. However, I highly recommend that you take proper lessons to ensure accurate, beneficial results.

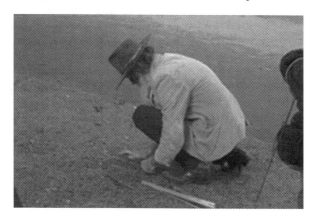

How Does Dowsing Work?

No one really understands why dowsing works, but there are several possible explanations. Some suggest there is an intuitive connection between the dowser and the information they are seeking. Since all things both living and inanimate give off energy, the dowser tunes into this field or vibration, which creates a response observed by the movement of the dowsing tool. Other explanations state our internal sensory systems are extremely sensitive to changes in the electrical and magnetic fields, which in turn cause involuntary movements of the muscles to occur. Some believe dowsing tools act as powerful antennas receiving information from vibrations produced by people, places, objects, and thoughts. But like many things we come in contact with daily, we do not necessarily need to understand why something works in order to use it. For example, even though people do not understand how electricity works, it does not stop them from turning on a power switch. Most individuals have no real understanding of how an automobile is able to get them from one place to another, yet this does not stop them from operating a motor vehicle. And although we cannot explain how a thought forms in our mind, it does not prevent us from thinking and communicating with one another. Some day we may have a clearer understanding of how dowsing works, but until then we can still benefit from utilizing this skill.

Dowsing is a fascinating practice, and if you find yourself desiring further information, please watch for a soon to be published booklet on Slim Spurling's dowsing techniques. For information on how to order this publication, please check the website **www.LightLifeTechnology.com**.

NOTES:

PART II
Improve Your Daily Life With The Light-Life™ Tools

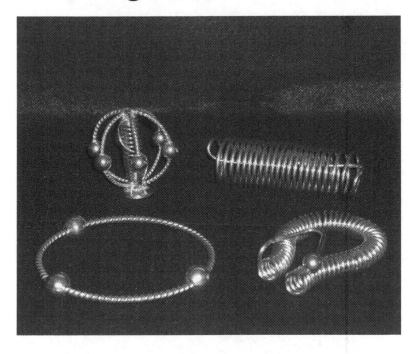

"The Light-Life Technology is an ancient science rediscovered to restore the health of the environment and mankind."

Slim Spurling

The Light-Life Tools and Technology came about as a result of years of study and research by Slim Spurling. To fully comprehend the tools, Part II opens with a chapter on key terms and principles that must be understood. Each subsequent chapter then covers an individual tool. These are presented in historical order of their development or their relationship to a previously designed tool.

Inside each chapter on the specific tools the following is included: background information, purpose, description, applications, and field reports. Field reports are from research associates who have purchased the tools. Most of these reports have been gathered by Slim and his wife Katharina Spurling-Kaffl. In addition, my husband, Scott, and I have submitted some of the field reports collected from individuals we have introduced the tools to.

It is here in Part II of the book where you'll read Slim's accounting of his discoveries, methods, and thoughts regarding his work. The material has been taken from various writings, articles, and transcripts of interviews by and of Slim Spurling.

What Are They Talking About? ~ Key Terms and Principles

This chapter contains the terminology and principles necessary to gain clear understanding of the Light-Life™ Technology created by Slim Spurling. Most of the information is provided directly from Slim himself through his interviews and writing.

KEY TERMS/PRINCIPLES

Light-Life™ Technology
Neter
Cubits
Cubit: Sacred
Cubit: Lost
Cubit: New
Sacred Geometry
Scalar Energy
Superconductivity
Tensor Field
Toroid
Vesica Piscis
Plating
Plain Jane

Light-Life Technology

In 1991, after years of research in the field of subtle energy, I developed a device now known as the Light-Life Ring. This ring was to become the prototype of a cutting edge technology.

The science represented in the ring technology is both ancient and modern. The Sacred Cubit length of 20.6 inches is the controlling factor in the construction. From the works of John Archibald Wheeler, the term "tensor" and its description as being formed when the ends of a piece of wire are joined in a loop, links the ring technology to modern advanced physics. At the time of Wheeler's writing in 1957, there was no known application for the tensor except as a mathematical theory. Myself, Bill Reid, and others discovered multiple applications for the energy field known as the tensor before reading Wheeler's work.

The current list of applications for the Light-Life Technology falls into several categories: air pollution control; health issues; stress reduction created by EMF and geopathic stress lines; water and soil treatment; agriculture; pest control; severe storm abatement; creating rainfall; and synergizing with other technologies.

The ring has evolved into several different tools through an empirical, intuitive, and experimental trial and error process. A second cubit length was discovered by Hans Becker in 2000 and incorporated in the technologies that same year. A third cubit was revealed to me by another gentleman in 2006, but I don't yet have the capacity to go into production with it.

A research association was formed to further discover new applications for the tools and share information with an international network. Ongoing research into the effects of the tools and their applications is being conducted with the assistance of renowned scientists, technicians, and qualified lay researchers.

Neter

The ancient measurements known as neter lengths are used in the construction of all our tools. Suffice it to say that the Ancients were better informed about the true nature of this reality than we are! Put simply, neters are "codes" for the specific wavelengths or frequency lengths that Spirit employs to manifest here in 3-D.

There are nineteen known neter lengths that have come down to us. More likely there are sixty-four, but so much ancient knowledge has been lost or hidden, nineteen are all we have to work with at this time. These measurements have been preserved in the structure of The Great Pyramid and in many of the sacred sites all around the world. They can also be extracted through a thorough study of the circumferential, radial, and diametric proportions of the earth. Each of these sacred measurements holds frequencies that embody different functions or qualities of Spirit. Note: Since the time when Slim spoke these words, Hans Becker discovered the Lost Cubit measurement, and another gentleman, the New Cubit measurement.

The quality of Spirit encoded in each neter length could be compared to the Spirit of God, or the male principle. The opening created when the two ends are joined together is analogous to the Great Void, or the female principle. When God spoke into the Great Void, or stirred the waters of the deep, and the male polarity united with the female polarity, it gave rise to The Word, or frequencies of sound. When The Word was spoken, and those sound frequencies began to vibrate, Light was generated.

As soon as these sacred measurements of twisted wire are soldered into a circle, the frequency or quality of Spirit inherent in each neter length begins to vibrate or sing across the center plane of every ring. Research has shown that the tensor field, or the empty space within the circumference, starts to vibrate at either 144 MHz or 177 MHz depending on which measurement is used. 144 MHz, which is associated with the Sacred Cubit, is a harmonic of the speed of light in free space. So this particular measurement has the properties of giving the rings a natural resonant frequency of 177 MHz. The fact that it vibrates faster than the speed of light is worthy of note. It is easy to assume that this would render it more powerful on some level.

This information alone would be enough to make anyone perk up and say, "Aha! Now I can see why there's something remarkable about these rings!" But there is more. The frequencies generated by the tensor effect are not confined to the ring opening. They actually form a beam or column of light that extends outward from the plane within the circumference of the wire, infinitely, in both directions! This beam holds and transmits higher light frequencies over a distance. Anything you aim a ring at, place it around, or put it on will be enlightened and uplifted by the energies pouring out of the tensor.

Cubit Measurements

The standard unit of linear measurement in ancient Egypt was the cubit. To ensure standardization of the cubit length, the Egyptians created a master measuring instrument carved out of granite containing notches identifying various subdivisions, of which the cubit length had twenty-eight. This was the criteria upon which all other cubit sticks were subsequently measured and calibrated. When a construction project such as erecting a temple, a pyramid, or a tomb was underway, cubit measuring rods were supplied to workers. The royal architect who was responsible for overseeing the construction project and maintaining the precise standards of measurement would issue granite or wooden cubit sticks to the workers. The sticks were required to be returned each full moon to be compared to the Pharaoh's master cubit stick. Severe penalties were enforced for failure to do so, resulting in death. "With this standardization and uniformity of length, the Egyptians achieved surprising accuracy. Thousands of workers engaged in building the Great Pyramid of Giza. Through the use of cubit sticks, they achieved an accuracy of 0.05%. In roughly 756 feet or 9,069.6 inches, they were within 4 ½ inches." (Bucher, Jay L.)

According to Slim, the cubit measurements *"are measurements taken from natural phenomenon and they're related to the structure of the earth, to the speed of light, to atomic weights, and atomic radii - that is, the difference between the nucleus in the electron orbits of hydrogen."*

Sacred Cubit

The Sacred Cubit was found in the pyramid at Giza, the Great Pyramid, and it's found as a unit of measurement in a yardstick in many areas of the ancient world. This particular measurement was carved in stone just above the entrance to the King's Chamber. That is the measurement of the perimeter of the boss - the little projection of stone just 72.1 inches above the floor of the King's Chamber. The cubit length is used throughout the measurement, throughout the pyramid.

[Note: The measurement of the boss is one Sacred Cubit equaling 20.6 inches. This is the measurement used for the 1 Sacred Cubit Ring. The measurement from the floor to the boss is 72.1 inches or 3.5 times the Sacred Cubit. This is the measurement used for the large ring, called the 3.5 Cubit Ring.]

The rings made in this cubit length have a natural resonant frequency of 144 MHz, which is a harmonic of light speed. In recent years, we've discovered that it is also a measurement of a wavelength in the standing gravity wave of the planet.

Now how do you measure gravity waves and how do you measure their wavelengths? The Ancients were able to do this, and in recent years, a gentleman named Hartmut Müller in Germany has developed mathematics to describe the full spectrum of gravity wave frequencies. And in that, he has discovered that this particular wavelength appears to be connected to the constructive phase of solid matter. Witness the fact that with his particular measurement, the Great Pyramid is the longest surviving structure on the planet. And of course, it was built by a civilization with a profound knowledge of mathematics, physics, astrophysics, and we believe, gravity - and the probability that they also used some kind of a levitational or antigravity system to build the pyramids, to lift the stones into place. That's yet to be duplicated in the modern world, as far as we know.

Lost Cubit

In 2000, a friend of mine, named Hans Becker, and I discovered another cubit length. He was looking for the measurement lying between the Sacred Cubit and the Royal Cubit, which is about 25.3 inches. There was a gap in the known sequence of different cubit lengths. So Hans got busy with his calculator one day and he took the polar circumference of earth, the equatorial circumference of earth, and divided that into the speed of light, and converted all of these measurements in feet, or miles, or miles per second into inches, then divided by two until it came down to a comfortably small number. And that is the "Lost Cubit," also called the Becker Cubit. The Lost Cubit measurement, a discovery of Hans Becker, is derived from the sum of the polar and equatorial circumferences of the earth, in inches, divided into the speed of light. The Lost Cubit is larger than the Sacred Cubit. In its relationship to the Sacred Cubit, it is like the atmosphere of the earth is to the diameter of the earth.

Also called the "Forbidden Cubit," this previously unknown cubit measurement is not recorded in the ancient texts, but it fills a harmonic gap between the established Sacred and Royal Cubits. As discussions progressed, the idea surfaced that all the knowledge relating to this measurement might have been deliberately hidden or lost. Truly transformative power is often kept back from the general audience and held in the hands of a chosen few.

Early professional reports point to effects consciously and willfully created when an intention is fueled by a strong emotional content felt within the researcher's physical body. As of late, what some healers are noticing is that the tensor field of the Lost Cubit functions much like a lens or a window, which allows them to view information that is stored in the Akashic records. When a Lost Cubit Ring is held over a client or chakra or problematic area, deeper knowledge appears to be transferred or picked up by the field inside the ring. It deals more with the atmosphere or aura of a person, there being an analogy, and it deals more with the mental and emotional issues we human beings experience. We find, often times, a release from long standing emotional or mental problems when using the Lost Cubit.

Cubit Length Comparison: Sacred vs. Lost

By comparison, the Sacred Cubit, the smaller of the two, defines the solid matter of earth. The Lost Cubit, being somewhat larger, would define the atmospheric frequencies of the planet. There's a spatial relationship between the two, which would look like a photograph of the earth from space with that very, very thin shell of atmosphere around it showing up as somewhat of a blue haze on that sharp horizon against the darkness of space.

One of the interesting things we found for the healers is that the Sacred Cubit, whether it's of the half cubit size or the one cubit size, seems to deal with physical problems very readily, whereas the Lost Cubit seems to deal more with mental and emotional problems or distortions in the aura. What we call problems are actually electrical or energetic distortions within the human aura. And so by comparing these, you can see that the smaller ring size can be equated to physical matter and the larger ring size can be equated to the aetheric, or the atmosphere of the human, or of any plant, or of any animal. I wanted to clarify that there is a distinct difference in the size and that their interaction can perhaps even provide some interesting highlights in terms of the energetic interaction of the two.

CHAPTER 6

New Cubit

In 2011, Katharina Spurling-Kaffl received a phone call from a gentleman who gave her a new cubit measurement for a ring. She made some prototypes of this ring and sent them to a research group for evaluation. After receiving feedback from the group, IX-EL, Inc. began manufacturing the ring. Katharina considers the New Cubit to be the final link in the trinity of cubit measurements. She has called the new ring the **Empowerment Ring,** as it seems to support mental clarity and activity as well as enhancing healing processes. The gentleman had given the measurement to Slim in 2006; however, Slim did not have the manufacturing capacity to make those rings at the time.

Sacred Geometry

Everything in existence is a structured pattern of creation. This includes the physical, from the smallest particle of matter through to the largest most magnificent objects found in the universe, and all aspects in between, both living and non-living. In addition, it encompasses that which exists on the other levels from the mental, emotional, and spiritual dimensions. Embedded in each structured pattern is a unique energetic vibration or frequency signature. The manner in which all of these vibratory frequencies interact with one another displays the fundamental unity of the part to the whole.

These patterns that surround us everywhere, permeating everything, can be referred to as sacred geometry, the vehicle through which Spirit enters and assimilates into matter. By replicating and then applying the geometry found in nature and in the movements of the cosmos to what we create, we facilitate bringing together the resonance of harmonic frequencies existing between the heavens and earth. It is through this process we begin to understand, demonstrate, and experience how everything is connected, thus creating a bridge between the dimensional worlds.

In sacred geometry, it is the belief that patterns and numbers have a divine or sacred meaning. Included in this group are some of the traditional geometric forms such as the sine wave, the sphere, the Vesica Piscis, the torus, the golden ratio, and the five platonic solids. Throughout history, many mystical and spiritual practices, such as astrology, Feng Shui, and geomancy began with an underlying adherence to the principles of sacred geometry. Today, architects, designers, musicians, scientists, and inventors can be counted among those that frequently incorporate the study of sacred geometry into their work. Thus, it is from this field the foundation for the construction of the Light-Life Technology lies in the utilization of the Sacred Cubit measurements.

The Sacred Cubit length was selected because of the particular frequency it holds of 144 MHz, and once this linear measurement was constructed into a circular form and connected, it created a column of light. Further study and experimentation lead to the discovery of the Lost Cubit measurement. "The Lost Cubit has a natural resonant frequency of 177 MHz which corresponds to the frequency of DNA, thereby facilitating DNA repair and the capability of consciously controlled DNA activation and ascension. It is becoming more widely accepted by scientists that DNA acts as an antenna for light energy and, therefore, the harmonic frequencies of light and the Lost Cubit, in particular, are vitally important aspects of the equation." (Beyond Energy Healing) Using the geometry of shape, form, ratios, and patterns, Slim Spurling was able to make discoveries that he then incorporated into the Light-Life Tools. These tools, in their various applications, help to make the space in which they are used more coherent and vital, while assisting in bringing about order and harmony.

SCALAR ENERGY

Scalar energy is not well known in the general scientific community. It's not part of the daily language in science classes at the university. Scalar energy is reserved for the elite of the elite in theoretical quantum physics. It's been known and described for many years. But the actual application of scalar energy has not been available to the public. And we didn't know what to call it or how it worked, to date. I mean, we CAN apply it, we can SEE results. The effect we see is rapid healing. With certain techniques, we can see broken bones heal in as little as an hour. An expert practitioner can heal a broken bone in ten minutes.

FURTHER EXPLANATION

Looking to find an easy to understand explanation of scalar energy that could be grasped by the layman without an extensive scientific background, I came across a helpful introductory article by Bill Morgan entitled, Scalar Energy – A Completely New World is Possible. He states, "Scalar energy is a new kind of electromagnetic wave, which exists only in the vacuum of empty space, the empty space between the atoms of our bodies, as well as the empty space we see in the sky at night. These waves constitute a kind of ocean of infinite energy, and it has now been discovered that this abundant energy can be coaxed to pour into our three-dimensional world from their four-dimensional realm, to be used to do work, provide electricity, power all transport, and even heal the body of almost all disease. This is the new world of scalar electromagnetics, the zero-point energy, and the energy of the absolute nothingness which existed before the world began."

SCALAR ENERGY - IS IT LIFE FORCE ENERGY?

It appears to be identical to the life force energy, the same chi energy that a skilled chi gong practitioner would use, or the hands-on healers. And I was able to find the relationship there probably within a week of the discovery of the rings back in 1991.

SUPERCONDUCTIVITY

A definition of superconductivity provided by Dr. Tom Lynch is "the flow of electric current without resistance in certain metals, alloys, and ceramics at temperatures near absolute zero and in some cases, at temperatures hundreds of degrees above absolute zero." (Superconductivity for Teachers)

Every ring is a superconductor. Research has shown that the light they generate expands the orbital radius of every electron lying in their path. This effect endows anything in that field to hold more energy and more light. The impact of these higher light frequencies acts to displace or transmute anything within their range that is not of the light. Thinking about this, it is easy to see why the rings have such positive healing properties.

We don't fully understand it yet, but we don't understand electricity either. We can run it through wires. We can project it across space. We can do a number of things with it. But this technology is much like the early days of electricity. It was a parlor game or a parlor experiment. And our early scientists, Michael Faraday and Galvani, were using simple devices, and now we're using simple devices again in this modern age. We know them to be superconductors. We know them to produce a naming system to be able to call this energy what it is or what it will be called. So, we're just saying it's a bio-energy and it is effective in restoring proper balance to the body.

TENSOR FIELD

The tensor is a term from quantum physics, so we are dealing with some sort of quantum effect, some kind of application of quantum physics to everyday life.

Later in our readings of advanced quantum physics, we found the term tensor reported by John Archibald Wheeler, who wrote a book in 1957 titled "Geometrodynamics," and he said any loop of wire creates a tensor, a field of energy. This is a mathematical calculation; it's called a minimal surface. So what his report was, if you dip this loop of wire in a soap solution like you are going to blow bubbles like every kid on the planet has done, that the soap solution is actually hanging on this tensor energy field. This is his description of the tensor. If you want to know what it looks like, dip it into soap and that's what you will see. Soap makes water wetter. It's what is called a surfactant, and the water shouldn't stick to anything as well. It penetrates better but it has less surface tension. It is the energy field itself supporting physical matter on nothing but a network or a film of pure energy that is created by the metal loop.

TOROID

Toroid is not a term I hear mentioned frequently. Actually, other than math class years ago and working with the Slim Spurling tools, I rarely encounter the word at all. So put in very simplistic terms, a toroid is a geometric shape. Picture the following images: a *smoke ring* from a cigar moving through the air, a child playing on the sidewalk with a *hula hoop*, someone getting ready to bite into a yummy glazed covered *doughnut,* or even you using a 1 Sacred Cubit *Ring*. Each of these images brought forth are examples of this shape. If the shape is hollow, like the examples of the smoke ring or hula hoop, it is referred to as a torus. On the other hand, if it is solid like the donut or ring, then it is called a toroid. So worded a bit differently, a torus is the surface area of a toroid, and the toroid is the form encased by a torus. It is a sphere shape that curves inward on top and bottom, having a hole in the center.

These forms are all around us. They are created by winding a circle around an axis that is external to the circle. You may be familiar with a toy called a Spirograph. The design created by this simple toy is formed by repeated circular rotations with each circle meeting at the center. This significance of the toroid shape is that it allows energy to spiral inwards and outwards on the same surface.

VESICA PISCIS

When two circles of the same size overlap through the center of one another sharing a common area, the Vesica Piscis is formed within that joined space. The meaning of Vesica Piscis is *Vessel of the Fish*, which contains many symbolic representations. "In ancient symbolism, it stood for the feminine creative force or mother-Spirit that gave birth to worlds and to the gods that maintained them." (Chandler, Wayne B). This symbol has been of significance through the ages, readily incorporated in various cultures, and used extensively in religion, art, architecture, and mathematics. It can be seen in logos, in building design, and as the basis for the Flower of Life. Some mystical symbolism included the unification of the male and female, the sign of fertility, and as the all-seeing eye leading to the window of the soul. The frequency in which this symbol appears across cultures illustrates the universal fascination we have as a society with ratios and proportions. The Vesica Piscis form has been integrated into a few of Slim Spurling's Light-Life Tools, such as in the design of the Seed of Life and the Lotus Pendant.

PLATING

Plating is the process of applying a thin coat or plate of a selected metal to a conductive surface. This technique has a long history going back to ancient times. Plating has been used for a variety of purposes: decorating objects, finishing jewelry, protecting against deterioration, improving soldering ability, hardening matter, reducing friction, modifying conductivity, enhancing the bonding of paint, and as a shielding element against radiation.

The original rings had no plating on them. After about a year of constructing rings, silver plating was applied. People inquired about the possibility of applying gold plating to the rings as well. This was not done until money was available to buy 24K gold solution. This solution was chosen because of its higher vibratory levels, speed, and smoothness of action. All plated Light-Life Tools have a layer of silver first, and then 24K gold plating. All Personal Harmonizers and pendants have at least eight or nine layers of alternating silver and gold. According to Slim, *This multi-layering creates a thermocouple effect. As a result, a small voltage is generated and converted instantly to amperage or current by all of the tools to increase the energy field. The tools and jewelry are not lacquered like commercial 24K gold plated jewelry. Due to the superconductive nature of all Light-Life Tools, the plating tends to sublimate. This gaseous state then is readily available in its diffuse nature to provide sub-micro trace nutrients to the body, aura, and environment, gradually raising the vibration of all.*

PLAIN JANE

The Plain Jane Ring is called this because it is made of copper, and it has no beads and no plating. Its natural tendency to oxidize with age gradually boosts the power of the ring. Copper oxide (CuO) is one of the first doping compounds used to boost the power and efficiency of computer chips.

Technically, copper oxide is a non-linear coating, which acts as an interface between the metal conductor and the aether energy of space. It is somewhat like a step-down transformer in its action, lowering the enormous potential of the "aetheric energies" to a useful and easily manageable level, while modulating the natural frequencies arriving from the cosmos.

CHAPTER 7

Energize Your Life with
The Light-Life™ Rings

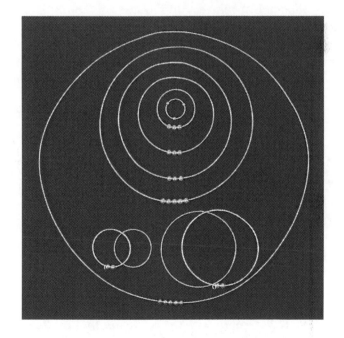

Pictured from Large – Small:
3½ Cubit – 2 Cubit – 1½ Cubit – 1 Cubit
– ½ Cubit – ¼ Cubit
(all in Sacred Cubit)

*"These discoveries are really rather remarkable. We have a
phenomenal technology which we're not at the end of exploring."*

Slim Spurling

BACKGROUND OF THE LIGHT-LIFE RINGS

I would like to begin with the discovery and development of the rings. These are very simple copper wire constructions. The active part of the ring is the open space. It's the unseen energy field. Occasionally with proper lighting and certain angles, you can see with normal vision a very thin sort of shimmering energy field in here that appears to reflect light or to generate light. We have ample evidence, both photographic and personal observations, of this energy field. This is called a tensor. The tensor is a term from quantum physics, so we're dealing with some sort of quantum effect, some kind of an application of quantum physics to everyday life.

The ring was discovered in 1991, as a result of a gentleman who came from Kansas to introduce his technology to the scientific community or anyone who would listen. He claimed to be able to heat or cool a building and reduce the heating and cooling bills. This could be done, he claimed, with a length of copper wire about three quarters of an inch in diameter, and a little over three feet long. So, he passed on this device to us, and one afternoon we were gathered, I believe there were five of us in the room, trying to understand how this thing worked. We used pendulums; we used electrical meters; we used any number of devices to attempt to identify this energy. In the middle of our discussion, we had a couple of clairvoyants drop in to visit. One of them suggested that we simply bring the ends of this cable together and clamp them. Well as we did that, the lady who was extremely clairvoyant jumped back like she'd been subjected to an electric shock. What had happened -- as the ends of that cable touched, she had seen a brilliant flash of light appear above the plane of the ring. So here's this heavy cable, the ends are brought together in a circle, the light appears above the ring, and she jumps back like she had been electrocuted.

After we got her calmed down, we proceeded to investigate this very carefully, and we were able to determine with the pendulum that there was an energy flow above the ring in the light field that she saw moving in a clock-wise direction. Underneath the ring, there was an energy field that she could not see with clairvoyant vision, but that energy field was moving in a counter clock-wise direction. And no matter if we were measuring with the pendulum hanging beneath the ring, or if we were measuring above the ring, it always moved counter clock-wise.

Later we discovered that a simple light gauge copper wire would have a similar effect, and we made a number of these, always being careful to identify the positive and negative side of the ring. In that process, we were just avoiding this negative side because we believed that it would have a negative effect. Very soon we had some accidents or incidents, which proved this. One of our co-researchers had been experiencing some heart problems, and we gave him a couple of rings and one of the early models of the coil. We could get some of the pain reduced that he was experiencing and he seemed to feel better. But in the overall, on a day to day average, he would be up and down; he would have more pain one day, and less pain the next.

So, one day he says, "I'm gonna fix this thing." He puts the negative side of the ring up to his heart and instantly his heart stopped beating. Well, in a couple minutes he hits the floor, and says, "Oops, I think I'd better turn it over." So he put the positive side toward his heart, and immediately the heart started beating again. He called us immediately and told us the story. We then collected all of these single wire rings that we'd produced because of the potential harm that MIGHT be done, and brought everything back to the shop, cut them up in little pieces and took them out of circulation.

PURPOSE OF THE LIGHT-LIFE RINGS

Everywhere we look we find success, and across a range of applications, that is absolutely staggering. Almost any human endeavor - in production of materials, in health care, in well-being, in preservation of food, plants, and so forth, will benefit. There's just an endless list.

DESCRIPTION OF THE LIGHT-LIFE RINGS

There are two factors: one is the measurement. We use the Sacred Cubit lengths for our measurements. The cubit lengths are taken from the Egyptian Pyramid, the Great Pyramid, and that is from the yardstick or the fundamental metric that was used in the pyramid. The Sacred Cubit length, which we measure in conventional inches, is 20.6 inches. The circumference of the ring then, is 20.6 inches, give or take a few hundredths. This measurement is probably, as we've recently learned, tied into the fundamental wavelength of a portion of the gravity field, which has to do with construction.

We all know how resonant frequencies can either create or destroy. We use the example of bridges collapsing when troops are all marching in unison. That can cause harmonics, which can cause a bridge to structurally disintegrate. What we found is this cubit length seems to cause things to integrate rather than disintegrate. The frequencies and energy field generated then resonate at the creation level of energy. If we move over here, we would probably find a different length, which could create or destroy structural materials. But we're not interested in that. We're only looking for beneficial effects.

It's the intrinsic nature of the measurement and the form of energy that we're using. So with the discovery of the on-powered caduceus winding, which just happens to be a superconductor at room temperature, and verified by laboratories and a number of different scientists, we now have the ability to create power, to create an energy field that has a very, very positive effect on a wide range of living and non-living materials.

We're talking about frequencies. Any length of wire would generate light or an energy field of a kind, or of the same kind, but the frequency would not be in the constructive or beneficial range. In other words, for instance, DNA is subject to electromagnetic radiation - cell towers, microwaves, all sorts of things. We don't particularly want to cook ourselves. But this is electromagnetic energy. The rings transduce or change the form of energy. A ring will, say, pick up radio waves, which are electromagnetic, and convert them to a different form of energy in the beam coming from the ring. So this is a transducer; it changes the energy.

Additionally, we found that the rings are perfect antennas for gravity field energies. And gravity field is universal. So, now we have the frequencies of the gravity field in addition. It appears that the rings are driven by the universe and all the contained frequencies in that composite. This is the culmination of over 20 years of research, my personal observations, and my scientific studies with other individuals, other scientists. And this is how we understand these tools now - that they are a culmination of all the power sources, not only of the planet, but they're driven also by the very power of the universe. And we see that through the gravitational field sensitivity of these tools.

I worked out the topology of the creation of this energy field, either positive or negative, and was able to develop a ring such as this current model, which has a positive energy field above it and a positive energy field below it. A good clairvoyant can see the energy field like a beam, a cylinder of light. So now we have a device, which has ONLY positive effects. As you look at the topology of a ring, in other words the way it's constructed, the ring is comprised of a single piece of wire. Now you look at it and say, Oh no, that's two pieces of wire, and if you look at the cut end sections of this twisted wire, indeed there are two pieces.

However, in the construction, the wire is stretched out, folded back on itself, twisted, and then cut to the appropriate length. Thus, it is actually one piece of wire. Now one of the interesting things that we know as dowsers is that any linear object has a plus and minus end or a north and south pole. Or you could look at it as a west and east pole. But there is a distinct difference in the way the pendulum rotates. So this is a ver significant thing, to be able to identify these ends, to bring the wire into a neutral state, which occurs when you join plus and minus. It becomes neutral right at the soldered joint.

CADUCEUS COIL WINDING AND CONNECTIONS TO THE RING WINDING

My partner, Bill Reid, and I started with a caduceus coil. We wrapped a piece of double strand lamp cord on a pure iron rod and hooked it up to a light bulb, or an old radio with a tuner on it, and projected a beam of energy out the end of the iron rod. We had read about this somewhere and had a crude drawing. We called a clairvoyant friend and she was able to tell us that there was definitely a beam coming out of the end. We experimented with many things.

Well, in this caduceus winding on the iron rod, the wire is wrapped down the length and then back over itself, which cancels the magnetic field. We found that there was no electrical or radio frequency detectable when this was in operation. There was, however, a slight magnetic field at the end of the rod simply because that's the nature of the iron. It has a polar nature. And it definitely had a magnetic function before and after winding that caduceus winding on it.

The clairvoyant sees the two energy fields as being identical. And we learned over the many years of research to trust the clairvoyant vision. It saves us, oftentimes, having to use the facilities of a multi-million dollar laboratory to determine polarity, to determine the direction of energy field flow. The size, the dimension, and even the color can be determined in an instant by a good clairvoyant. And, oddly enough, many, many of the scientific laboratories actually rely on clairvoyants.

The Caduceus Coil Rod Applied to Water

We put the caduceus beam in a pint of water and precipitated out a great number of different minerals. Using Denver, Colorado, tap water we got copper, silver, gold, mercury, and other metals we didn't identify, and also what looked like sand.

We noticed the metals and minerals were falling out of the water. I started drinking a half a glass a day spread over several sips. You always start carefully with new things, especially dealing with subtle energy. One of the things we noticed was an increase in our energy levels, our mental clarity, and a general feeling of well-being. So, in this process we began to use more and more of it.

During a single two to three week period, Bill Reid and I were doing some extremely heavy labor in July heat and no wind out there, so I just brought a gallon of this water along and used that entirely for drinking water. And so in the course of one day, I'd consumed an entire gallon of water. The net effect was an enormous detox, a flushing of the entire system. To be very blunt, there was a flush of a diarrhea. It was very discolored, very odorous, and this was a result of drinking an entire gallon, and flushing all these toxins out of the system through normal elimination. This is very often experienced, not to that degree, but it can be experienced by anyone who begins experimenting with these tools. It can be a mild detox if you use a little bit and slowly increase over time, but I don't recommend drinking an entire gallon of potentized water in a single day.

Potentized Water

We had a number of individuals with various ailments that had been medically diagnosed, and they were willing to experiment with potentized water. Universally, they experienced the benefits of having more energy, less pain, less discomfort, and in some cases, a complete disappearance of symptoms. I recall one individual, a powerful attorney in Denver, who drank over the course of six months something in the neighborhood of 15-20 gallons of potentized water produced with this caduceus coil, and his symptoms completely disappeared.

MAKING POTENTIZED WATER

This little caduceus winding on this rod only produced a pencil-sized beam. And we'd project that beam through a gallon of water, or five or six gallons of water even, and it would take 8, 10, or even 12 hours to reach its maximum potency.

It was frustrating not to be able to produce enough to be able to put it in the hands of the people. I'm a firm believer that everyone should have the ability to do whatever is necessary for their own personal health and well-being. It may take a little training, a little experience, but it's available to everyone.

So I'm looking at this pencil-sized beam and I'm saying, "we've got to find a better way to do it." Well, when we discovered the ring, I mean, this was like an answer to prayer. This does not use any electrical power whatsoever and produces what is called gravity field energy. Energizing a gallon of water with these new rings was instantaneous!

Now we have a cross-section in any size we want; it can be as small as an inch in diameter, as large as six inches in diameter, and we can go on up to a couple of feet in diameter, large enough to fit around the entire body. And that means an energy beam can be created in which an individual can stand, or plants and food can be placed. But, goodness sakes, this for me is freedom – to have in hand a remedy that works on this subtle energy level.

HOW A RING POTENTIZES WATER ~ OBSERVATIONS OF WATER TREATED WITH LIGHT-LIFE TECHNOLOGY

A Light-Life Ring increases the available energy in the water instantaneously. It causes water to emit light and it causes an expansion of the atomic radius. Now this is a deductive process. The way we came to this was through the use of an instrument, which would detect the change or increase in the available light being emitted from water. In other words, water has a certain level of energy as it sits in the glass, or exists in your water pipes, or a lake or stream.

What we found is that the rings cause an increase in energy, which manifests as an increase in full spectrum light all the way from infrared on up to ultra violet. But the increase in light energy can only occur if the electron orbit expands, rotates at a greater distance from the nucleus, and then falls back slightly to the next energy level. And when it falls back to the next energy level, it emits a photon. So, here's this little bitty energy package we call an atom with electrons whirling around it. They encounter the energy field of the ring. That expands; the electrons have a larger orbit. They fall back to their natural state and emit energy in the form of light.

The quantum effects have been studied instrumentally including spectral output of light from treated water in growth studies and taste tests, and verified or confirmed by psychic observation. The light field imparts "livingness" to water, which enhances the "life force" when consumed or used to water plants or animals. Water changes from very acidic pH to neutral or slightly alkaline when left standing in the ring for 24-48 hours. Taste tests show that water treated with a ring is softer, cleaner, and feels purer than untreated water.

The surface tension of water is lower when a container of it is set momentarily in the light field, or the ring is held over the container. Treated water has a lower freezing point and a different crystalline structure than the ice of untreated water. Take two identical glasses of water with ice cubes at your lunch table, set one in a ring, the other a foot or so away, and see which melts first!

Psychics and radionics operators verify greater 'vitality' of water. The rings cause water to fluoresce. These quantum light effects have been studied instrumentally and confirmed through psychic observation. The 'light' field above or below the ring appears to relax the cell membranes to allow better oxygen/nutrient/waste transport in and out of the cell.

Katharina, myself, and a friend of mine met with Philip Callahan, author of "Paramagnetism: Rediscovering Nature's Secret" in December 2000. We gave Philip a few Light-Life Rings and an Agricultural Harmonizer. Later he later reported that he was very excited about his findings, which indicated the paramagnetic value of the Light-Life Tools was 18,000. This value is significant because it's six times greater than that of the highest naturally paramagnetic elements known! A paramagnetic element is one that has unpaired electrons. Aluminum is one example, as is oxygen.

SACRED CUBIT

The Sacred Cubit is taken from the pyramid and is the measurement of the perimeter of the boss, the little projection of stone 72.1 inches above the floor of the King's Chamber. The cubit length measurement is used throughout the pyramid. It's a standard unit like a foot or a yard, but in British inches, it measures 20.6 inches. The 1 Sacred Cubit has a natural resonant frequency of 144 MHz, which is a harmonic of light speed. In practice, the Sacred Cubit deals more with physical matter, although the atmosphere is physical and consists of molecules that are not solid necessarily, but have a solid physical basis.

LOST CUBIT

The Lost Cubit is larger than the Sacred Cubit. In its relationship to the Sacred Cubit, it is like the atmosphere of the earth is to the diameter of the earth. The 1 Lost Cubit has a natural resonant frequency of 177 MHz. It deals more with the atmosphere or aura of a person, there being an analogy, and with the mental and emotional issues we human beings experience. We often times find a release from long-standing emotional or mental problems when using the Lost Cubit.

NEW CUBIT

A final link in a trinity of cubit measurements, the New Cubit is a recently revealed measurement given to Katharina Spurling-Kaffl by a gentleman who was in communication with Slim before his passing. When Slim and this gentleman talked, Slim did not have the manufacturing capacity at the time to make rings of this size. This gentleman kept his promise to Slim not to make the rings himself for commercial use and conveyed the information to Katharina in late 2011.

RING MATERIALS

The rings are constructed from copper or sterling silver, then may be plated with a combination of silver and gold. *In addition, we add either audio or electronic frequencies known to produce healing effects and to have beneficial qualities. And that's encoded right into the copper on every single item we produce.* The following is a list summarizing some of the basic aspects of these materials as applied to the rings.

Copper

- Is the no frills, utilitarian ring
- Has no plating
- Best material for continual outdoor use; they may corrode, but their function is not affected.
- May or may not include beads
- Plain Jane: does not include any beads

Copper, Plated with Precious Metals

- With the gold plated rings, the base is copper, followed with a layer of silver plating, then 24K gold plating
- With the silver plated rings, the base is copper, followed with a layer of silver plating, then a layer of 24K gold plating, and finally, a second layer of silver plating

24K gold plating adds a higher frequency due to the structure of the 24K gold atom in the crystal as it's deposited onto these rings. Every 24K gold plated tool is first plated with silver.

Sterling Silver

- Pure sterling silver, not plated
- Standard sterling silver wire rings include two beads
- Heavy sterling silver wire rings do not have any beads
- A small labeling ring is added to designate as sterling silver and not silver plated

The sterling silver tools seem to work at a slightly different subtle level and they seem to be smoother and faster in operation. Smoother and faster won't mean anything to the reader right now, but those who are in daily practice and have worked with the tools for some time – chiropractors, MDs, massage therapists, and other healers – seem to have a preference for the action of the sterling silver. Yet, anyone – attorneys, bus drivers, housewives, laboring people – will get along just fine with the standard copper and gold plated tools, which are just as effective in the long run.

The 1 Sacred Cubit sterling silver Light-Life Ring was conceived as a farewell commemorative for the end of the Second Millennium. The two silver beads mark that passing. The sterling represents the shining achievements of our human race in the past 1000 years and acknowledges the base metal alloy that gives sterling its qualities.

Silver is a superior electrical conductor, handling greater voltages and currents in electric circuitry. Observationally, it has been seen to affect a somewhat stronger and smoother acting field of energy than plain copper, likely due to finer, higher frequency vibration. Functionally, several practitioners have reported more rapid improvement, shorter necessary sessions, and longer lasting results with clients having difficult problems.

The sterling silver rings may be optionally 24K gold plated to at least partially avoid the normal silver oxidation, and add an even higher vibration yet.

STERLING SILVER WITH 24K GOLD PLATING

- Base is sterling silver, followed by 24K gold plating.

24K gold plating adds a higher frequency due to the structure of the 24K gold atom in the crystal as it's deposited onto these rings.

RINGS WITHOUT BEADS

Rings without beads are used mainly in field applications, such as agriculture or gardening, or for putting on waterlines to generally improve the quality of water for plants or animals or ourselves. We also use these rings to reduce fatigue and stiffness on long road trips by sitting on them.

Rings with Beads

The beads are simply amplifiers. They add a bit of electrical energy, which is then converted from voltage to current. And that increases the strength and density of the field. This spherical capacitor was used by Tesla in the production of some of his free energy devices and energy transmission systems. We adapted that to our purpose, and what it does is just give the rings a little bit more horsepower. So, that's the purpose of the beads.

Heavy Gauge Wire

If we use a heavier gauge wire in the same diameter, it simply means that we have a greater field density. It's a stronger effect. And that would mean there's more light coming out and more energy, since we're using the same basic cubit lengths in both rings.

The practitioners tell us that they really like the heavier gauge rings for that reason. They're more effective. These thinner gauge rings will do a marvelous job over time. And we've added the beads to them to amplify the effects somewhat. There's just a heft to the heavier gauge rings that feels good. Many people choose them on that basis and intuitively feel there's a greater field strength there, which, in fact, there is. So whether it's the so-called Royal or Sacred Cubit or the Lost Cubit that we use here, the heavier gauge wire is just more effective.

Ring Dimensions

The rings are produced in several gauges of wire, from the ½ cubit to the 3½ cubit. The listing below shows the ring sizes and the diameter of the tensor field. The following measurements are close approximations of actual diameters to give you an idea of their size, but the true diameters may differ by a few hundredths of an inch.

½ Cubit Rings

Sacred: 3.5"/8.9 cm diameter
Lost: 4.0"/10.2 cm diameter

New: 4.2"/10.7 cm diameter

1 CUBIT RINGS

Sacred: 6.5"/16.5 cm diameter Heavy Wire: 6.0"/15.2 cm diameter
Lost: 7.5"/19.1 cm diameter Heavy Wire: 7.0"/17.8 cm diameter
New: 8.5"/21.6 cm diameter

1½ CUBIT RINGS

Sacred: 10.0"/25.4 cm diameter Heavy Wire: 9.7"/24.6 cm diameter
Lost: 11.2"/28.4 cm diameter Heavy Wire: 11.0"/27.9 cm diameter
New: 12.7"/32.3 cm diameter

2 CUBIT RINGS

Sacred: 13.2"/33.5 cm diameter Heavy Wire: 13.0"/33.0 cm diameter
Lost: 15.0"/38.1 cm diameter Heavy Wire: 14.7"/37.3 cm diameter
New: 17.0"/43.2 cm diameter

3½ CUBIT RINGS

Sacred: 23.5"/59.7 cm diameter Heavy Wire: 23.0"/58.4 cm diameter
Lost: 26.2"/66.5 cm diameter Heavy Wire: 26.0"/66.0 cm diameter
New: 30.0"/76.2 cm diameter

All measurements are approximate.

APPLICATION OF THE LIGHT-LIFE RINGS

There are many applications, from the obvious things of being able to change water and neutralizing odors, to relieving pain and discomfort without any physical manipulation, massage, or other physical intervention.

- *Less is better. In drinking potentized water, start with half a glass twice daily, and slowly increase over a week or two. Detoxification may occur, manifesting as dark urine, diarrhea, and rashes or pustules on the skin depending on the type and level of toxicity.*

Take it slow so as not to overload the eliminatory organs. Detoxing too rapidly may produce unpleasant symptoms.

- *Plants appear to grow more lushly, are taller, have larger leaves, and fewer insects and pests. Animals prefer ring treated water.*

- *The light from the ring penetrates everything in its path. Since the human body is about 70-80% water, this light goes deep into the cells, generating positive healing effects at the cellular level. The rings appear to relax the cell membranes and allow for better oxygen/ nutrient/ waste transport in and out of the cells.*

- *Healers will notice that the rings amplify their natural abilities making it possible to give more benefit to more people in less time. Healing sessions that normally take two hours without the ring, may only take between 10 - 45 minutes with the rings. Chakra clearing is also greatly enhanced by the rings.*

Note from Katharina Spurling-Kaffl: It seems that healing sessions do not take as long as they used to. Be observant as to the needs of each client. Be aware that the tools seem to adjust to the changes of the earth's energies and may speed up a healing session.

- *Hanging a large ring on the headboard in alignment with the body while asleep has a curative impact and produces beneficial sleep patterns. People report enhanced dream states, a need for less sleep, and wake up feeling refreshed and alive. Any configuration of rings placed under the mattress or under the bed alleviates chronic pain and, in some cases, has produced miraculous healing effects.*

- *Standing or sitting in the ring field while working or meditating increases energy and clarity levels.*

- *The beam effect makes it possible to do healing work at a distance.*

- *Aiming the beam of a ring perpendicular to the plane at storm clouds as a tornado or severe storm approaches, reduces the severity of impact and, in some situations, will make threatening weather patterns disappear altogether. Only use on clouds that exhibit a gray-green color, as this is a sign of hail or a harmful storm.*

- *Some people have found that the rings are helpful in releasing the negative effects of the electromagnetic fields of electric meters.*

MEDITATION

- The Sacred Cubit Ring was first used in meditation. Sitting on a 1 Sacred Cubit Ring has a noticeable effect in shortening the time required to achieve a meditative state, calming and centering the mind. Sitting in a 3½ Sacred or Lost Cubit Ring has the same effect, with an added whole body relaxing quality.

WATER USES

- *A jug of water set on a Sacred Cubit Ring quickly loses its chlorine smell (two - three hours and appears much clearer and brighter than an identical jug not set on a ring. Start with ½ glass one to three times per day, as a detoxing effect may be noticed. As tolerance for the detoxing increases after several days, increase the intake. A general sense of more energy, reduced appetite, and less sleep needed usually occurs by the end of the second week. Some very brave souls have reported drinking a gallon a day from the start with rapid but not unpleasant detoxing, and energy levels not experienced since youth.*

- *Animals universally prefer Sacred Cubit Ring enhanced water to tap water. A birdbath filled with ring treated water needs to be refilled twice to three times a day to meet the demand from hordes of birds.*

- *A sunburn is quickly relieved by spraying or soaking a wet compress with Sacred Cubit Ring enhanced water.*

- *Sacred Cubit Rings on water faucets and showerheads reduce soap needs, and the morning shower is significantly more invigorating. Try with and without a ring for a few days.*

- *A Sacred Cubit Ring on the garden hose for lawn and garden application will reduce watering requirements and increase plant vigor and yield. We have seen aphids disappear from roses overnight when lightly sprayed.*

- *A large commercial vegetable farming operation in New Zealand was saved from bankruptcy when Sacred Cubit Rings were applied to irrigation pipes, ditches, and sprinklers resulting in a 30% increase in yield and a great increase in quality. The export buyers are paying in advance for these higher quality veggies because they arrive in fresher condition at distant ports in Japan and Europe with little appreciable deterioration and are free of insect, bacterial, and viral pests.*

RELAXATION/SLEEP

- Dogs and cats will often seek out and sleep in or on a 3½ Sacred Cubit Ring left on the floor.
- A 3½ Sacred Cubit Ring under the mattress has relieved chronic back spasm and sleeplessness.
- *Sitting on a 1 Sacred Cubit Ring on an airline trip, especially for intercontinental flights, significantly reduces jetlag for most travelers.*
- A 3½ Sacred Cubit Ring around an emotionally stressed individual helps to restore their composure.
- *Sleep with a 1 Sacred Cubit Ring under your pillow to help induce a good night's sleep. This also has, at times, the additional benefit of producing some very vivid dreams.*

SENSORY IMPROVEMENT

- *Voice quality and information transfer to an audience is significantly improved speaking through a Sacred Cubit Ring. May look funny, but it works!*
- *Musical instruments achieve a fuller expression of their resonant frequencies, which has an appreciable effect on the audience and performer alike.*
- *Sacred Cubit Rings placed in front of stereo speakers generate a better than live performance quality to sound.*

REMOTE VIEWING

- *Psychics report a much improved clarity of perception when holding a Sacred Cubit Ring in front of their face and directing the "beam" toward the client at a distance. Some psychics are using the Lost Cubit Ring for the same purpose and have stunning results.*

COMPUTER USES/ELECTRONICS

- A ½ Sacred Cubit Ring under the computer keyboard or worn on the left arm dramatically reduces "computer burnout" in the user.
- A ½ Sacred Cubit Ring over the mouse relaxes the hand working with the mouse.
- *A 3½ Sacred Cubit Ring around the computer monitor helps contain EMFs coming off the screen.*
- Place a ½ or 1 Sacred Cubit Ring over the telephone or receiver cord to reduce interference. Place a set of Phone Rings on both your wireless and cell phones.
- *Place a 1 Sacred Cubit Ring over a wireless router to contain the RF energy (radio frequency).*

PERSONAL AND SELF CARE

- We have several reports that stiff wrists and shoulders relaxed and pain disappeared in a few hours with a Sacred Cubit Ring around the offending area.
- Numerous people have reported that certain types of headaches were gone in a few minutes wearing a 1 Sacred Cubit Ring on the head.
- Passing a 3½ Sacred or Lost Cubit Ring around the body, top to bottom, several times is very energizing first thing in the morning or when tired later in the day.
- A ½ Sacred Cubit Ring placed over an area of pain, irritation, or achiness helps to relieve the discomfort.

- Keep a ½ Sacred Cubit Ring in your pocket so it can be used at any time to treat a beverage. My husband always has one with him, and if he stops to get a drink at the local pub, he treats his beer by placing the ½ Sacred Cubit Ring around the glass. The bartender refers to it as "bar jewelry."

CLOTHING/SOFT GOODS

- *Static is quickly removed from clothing passed two to three times through a Sacred Cubit Ring. It also removes the "energy" of whoever had been wearing the garment previously.*
- *Shoes and leather goods feel softer when set in a 3½ Sacred Cubit Ring overnight.*
- *A 3½ Sacred Cubit Ring hung at the end of the closet makes all the clothing feel "alive."*
- *One person marketing dancewear passes every new item through a 3½ Sacred Cubit Ring before displaying, then scans the racks every evening to "freshen" after a day's handling. Her sales took a big jump and remain higher than the previous three-year average.*

HOLISTIC PRACTITIONER USES/WORKING WITH CLIENTS

- *A 3½ Sacred Cubit Ring is placed under the massage table to help relax the client.*
- *Place three to five 3½ Sacred Cubit Rings overlapped to form a Vesica Piscis under a massage table to facilitate the complete relaxation of the client.*
- *Different sizes of Sacred and/or Lost Cubit Rings are placed on the body during an energy healing session to help rebalance chi.*
- *A 3½ Sacred Cubit Ring is used at the completion of a body work session as part of the closing technique. The auric field is smoothed and balanced as the ring is gently swept over the client.*

- A 1 Sacred Cubit and/or 1 Lost Cubit Ring can be placed under the head of a client who is feeling stressed. Doing so will help to quickly relax him or her into the session.
- Placing a ½ Sacred Cubit and/or Lost Ring on each arm helps energize a practitioner during a healing session.
- *After a healing session, it is helpful to clear out the energy before the next client arrives. This can be done by walking around the room holding a 3½ Sacred Cubit Ring as you clear the air.*

FOOD AND SUPPLEMENTS/HOMEOPATHICS/ MEDICATIONS

- *Food is set inside a Sacred Cubit Ring on the counter to keep it fresh.*
- Place a 3½ Sacred Cubit Ring on top of your refrigerator to keep the contents of the freezer and refrigerator fresh.
- Place a 3½ Sacred Cubit Ring in the trunk of your car to energize the groceries on your way home from the market.
- Herbs and vitamin supplements are placed inside a Sacred Cubit Ring to keep them energized.
- Medication is placed inside a ring to help increase beneficial actions and decrease side effects. Do not put your homeopathic remedies inside a Sacred Cubit Ring because it may change their potency.

MISCELLANEOUS

- *Placing a ½ Sacred Cubit Ring around the gas tank spout may help to energize the gas entering the vehicle. Individuals have reported as much as 10 - 30% better gas mileage for regular gas.*

FIELD REPORTS FROM RESEARCH ASSOCIATES

Ring Technology in the Classroom (Names have been Changed)

"I was so excited when Sarah L. called me this afternoon to tell me of your wonderful offer for the kids at our school. I was dancing around the room.

"We've been keeping good track of this particular class since the beginning of the year. Ann D. has declared this is the worst class she has ever had in over 25 years of teaching Special Education. And, I'm afraid it's known by too many people at school as *The Class from Hell.* We now have four adults in the classroom fulltime and one teenage girl who comes in to help after lunch. In this group of eleven fourth and fifth graders, we have a little bit of everything. Some of the children have ADD, some ADHD; six of the children are autistic. None of them can work as a class or in small groups without fighting, and on a number of days we have had to create rotating stations so that each child works alone.

"Some of the children like to yell and scream for long periods of time. Shout-outs take place hourly, and we have two time-out desks on opposite sides of the room because one wasn't enough. In fact, sometimes we also have one on the floor behind Ann's desk.

"About three weeks before Christmas break, I took my 3½ Sacred Cubit Ring and the Acu-Vac Coil to school with me. I cleared a space on my desk for them, and just used the coil undetected for the first week, aiming it at the loudest or most disruptive of the children. Sometimes it was in constant motion!

"The second week the tools were at school, Tom, a high-functioning autistic fifth grade boy, was getting frustrated because he couldn't figure how to do the subtraction lessons the other students were getting as they came to the board. He couldn't figure out how to borrow. I worked with him for a few moments and saw that he was about to go into his routine where he screams, makes other noises, and throws himself on the floor. I told him to stop, and I held the coil in front of him and told him it was going to suck the confusion right out of him. He stopped because he was curious and watched as I held the coil to his forehead. After a minute or two, I asked him if there was any other place in his head that felt stuffed up and confused. He took the coil and moved it around his head to a couple of other places and told me it was sucking out all the bad stuff. Then he said he was ready to try again. I explained the process to him again and he got it. He was so excited, and when he was called, was able to go to the board and write the correct answer.

"After that, he couldn't stay away from the tools. He'd come to my desk, run the ring over his body a time or two, or ask me to, and then he'd say, "I think I need to use the coil for a minute." Soon he was using the ring on the other kids, asking if they needed to feel better. By this time, everyone had gotten interested in the tools. They discovered that the coil could take the pain out of anything from a hangnail to a bruised leg and hip. I was having trouble using it to quiet down loud children because it was always in use somewhere else.

"The week before Christmas vacation the children were so revved up they couldn't concentrate on anything. One student, John, was having one of his prolonged and loud crying fits – inside his backpack! When he was sent to time-out, he quietly went to the coat rack, emptied his backpack, took it to the time-out desk (a time-out is five minutes or less), and proceeded to have a twenty-minute crying fit, then chose to stay there for another ten minutes after he finished. We have a video of him the week before where he had his crying fit outside. Then he managed to find an empty cardboard box, which he put over his head and wailed all through recess and beyond. When the principal saw him she asked, "Where can I get a box?" It was that kind of week.

"John goes to time-out feeling like the world is against him and positive that we all hate him. He says no one understands him, he's sure he didn't do anything wrong, no one likes him, everyone is mean to him, he doesn't have any friends, etc., and my favorite, "You people just don't understand me!" Once he gets started, he's rolling for twenty minutes at least. Ann asked the district psychologist what is happening with him, as he is the sickest child she's ever seen in the self-loathing and depressed department. The psychologist told her that this self-pity is like a drug to him that fills receptor sites throughout his entire body, and it's become like an addiction to him.

"So on the Monday of the last week before Christmas break as he was passing my desk to go to the time-out seat, I called him aside just as he was ready to start one of his "poor me" tirades and showed him a gingerbread boy I was drawing. I took my pencil point and put dots all over it. I said, "This is you John." I continued to make dots and asked him if he noticed that once he got started feeling sad he couldn't stop. He said yes. I told him that when he did that the sadness rushed all over his body and filled all these little spots with sadness so that he felt bad all day, but that he could take the coil and suck it all out so he wouldn't have to feel bad.

"He took it, and it was the very first time-out he ever had where he was quiet. At the end of five minutes he handed it back to me and said he felt better. Now, this usually occurred two or three times a day. But all week he was able to catch himself before it flooded his body. Sometimes he used the coil, and sometimes he didn't. He even was able to play foursquare with the "regular" kids without blowing it. Usually he has a loud fit because he says they're trying to get him out when, actually, they do it to everybody. We were amazed all week waiting for him to ignite, but it didn't happen, and he even helped another classmate and found a friend. Usually these children don't help others because they're so needy themselves. School starts again on Tuesday, and I wonder how he's done in the last two weeks over Christmas vacation.

"I got Sarah L. excited about the work and she hasn't even seen the DVD yet. There are twelve kids in her class, third and fourth graders. We have one more special education teacher at school that we'll approach when school starts, and I know a couple of regular education fifth grade teachers who have a couple of trouble-makers in their classes that they may be willing to track.

"The building we are in is old, full of mold, and has horrible energy walls running all through it, especially our room. We also have no opening windows. It will probably be torn down this summer. I was going to teach the kids to dowse and correct the bad energy lines that run all through the room. Will I still need to do that if the Harmonizer is working? I'll probably teach them anyway so that they can test their bedrooms at home, but I'm curious about that.

"Oh, one last thing. When we were exchanging Christmas gifts the Friday before school let out, I discovered that the aides had bought me a six-inch ring. That was the biggest thing yet with the kids. Every child wanted to wear it on their heads, so we had to set the timer for five minutes to allow everyone a turn. Then Tom brought it over and put it on my head saying, "I think you need a turn too."

"I can't thank you enough! I also can't wait to see what happens as we begin to use the Harmonizer. So I'll say Happy New Year, and Many, Many Blessings to you both." *M.F., CA*

COMMENTS FROM SPECIAL EDUCATION ELEMENTARY SCHOOL STUDENTS

- "Slim Spurling invented the rings. The rings are one cubit long. He found out that the cubit measurement was over the door at the King's Chamber of the Great Pyramid in Egypt, so he decided to use it. Slim is a botanist and a blacksmith, so he makes the rings himself."

- "Sometimes we wear the rings on our necks, heads, arms, and sometimes, feet. They make us feel smart."

- "The first time I put it on, it made me feel happy and drained out all my un-listening energy. It makes you feel good."

- "When I first wore them, I felt like listening."

- "The first time I put them on, it felt like the mean things came out and the nice things came in."

PEACEFUL RELIEF

"I have to share the experience I had with the large Sacred and Lost Cubit heavy Light-Life Rings at a funeral. My brother-in-law had collapsed in his bathroom and died suddenly. After his service, I gave the widow, my husband's sister, an "aura shower" with my large 3½ Sacred and Lost Cubit Rings. She was standing and I took the ring, held it over her head and moved it slowly down to her feet, and then placed it on the floor. I took the other ring and did the same thing. I had her lay down on the bed, and I used the Magnum Feedback Loop and scanned her whole body. The change in her was so surprising. My husband, who was observing, and quite frankly didn't know much about the Light-Life tools, was amazed. His sister's face showed a glow and happy expression. Her shock at losing her husband so suddenly was replaced with a peaceful understanding that he was in a better place. Their other siblings also commented on the positive changes they saw.

"I also did an aura shower on her son. He noticed that his shoulders dropped about one inch when the weight of his father's sudden death was removed.

"I signed up for a support group that helps grieving people, and I hope to be able to comfort more people with the Light-Life tools. Thank you so much." *P.B., Germany*

HOW LIGHT-LIFE™ TECHNOLOGY AFFECTS WINE

Well, we're not going to convert water into wine, but by placing a glass or bottle of wine inside a ring, we can take very, very cheap wine and make it of a superior quality. And with this technique, the longer it sits, the better it gets. A week sitting in a ring just does marvels. But even short term, just passing a ring up and down over a glass of wine a few times makes a huge difference. Takes the bite out of it. Makes it more mellow.

THE RINGS AND WELL WATER

The ring will give good service on natural waters when installed over the wellhead and on the lines. For some improvement in city waters, use a ½ or 1 Sacred Cubit Ring on the main and branch lines. I know that the hardness will improve, as it has been shown in water lab tests that calcium is at least partially converted to magnesium (transmutation). Rings installed on a wellhead and lines at a 40-horse barn in Eagle, Colorado, resulted in a 70% reduction in vet expenses and a calmer, less aggressive bunch of horses.

RINGS HELP A PAINFUL BACK

"My spine is moderately curved in the shape of an "S" which has caused me discomfort and slight physical limitations. After attending a Light-

Life workshop and learning some of the many possible uses for their rings, I brought home several of the 3 ½ Sacred Cubit (standard light gauge) versions. I placed three of them in the Vesica Piscis arrangement between my mattress and box spring and immediately noticed a huge improvement in my back. My spine didn't suddenly become arrow straight or anything, but the very first morning after sleeping over them I felt much better. My usual 15 minutes of painful back-stretching exercises were completely unnecessary (and painless!) and I didn't make that "old man grunt" whenever I had to pick up something off the ground. It's actually easy to forget how uncomfortable I was because I have felt consistently better since that day.

"My wife has one placed so that her head is inside the projected energy field when she sleeps. She tells me that her dreams are more tranquil and she no longer suffers from vivid nightmares as she used to.

"I have another placed around the chair at my computer desk. My cat, who used to go behind my computer tower where she enjoyed the warm air while messing up all the wiring, no longer sets foot back there. Instead, she lays contentedly under the chair basking in the Light-Life energy field." *R.N., CO*

½ SACRED CUBIT RING

"A couple of years ago I had a bad fall on my knee. I used various remedies and healing meditations, and it healed fairly quickly. Recently, I woke up with much internal pain in the same knee. I did my healing meditations and then pinned the ½ Sacred Cubit Ring to a pair of leggings and wore it for seven to eight hours. Needless to say, after four to five hours, the pain had completely disappeared and has not been back since." *Anonymous*

2 SACRED CUBIT RING

"I treated a mother whose 16-year-old daughter had been diagnosed with cancer. This woman had a history of stress related stomach problems, such as pain, nausea, loss of appetite, etc. These problems occurred during her daughter's illness and surgery. She began sleeping with a 2 Cubit Ring over her stomach whenever she was uncomfortable. She

reported immediate and consistent relief for the first time in her life."
A.A., IL

1½ Lost Cubit Ring

"Our 11-year-old yellow lab had a small cyst on his lower eyelid for the past year. Our vet said it could be removed, but it would be very involved and they would also have to take part of his eyelid. Since it didn't seem to hurt him, we decided to leave it alone. A while ago, we put a 1½ Lost Cubit Ring on his neck. Within a month, the cyst dried up and dropped off." *S.B., MN*

Potentized Water

"I just want you to know that your products may be helping to save my life. I experience electromagnetic hypersensitivity syndrome, so exposure to geopathic stress and EMR can cause me more pain than most. There is definitely a rejuvenating quality to the potentized water. I experience a vibration throughout my body when I consume it." *A.H., IN*

Float Tank Experience

"I have been operating Blue Light Floatation here in NYC continuously since 1985. Since adding the 3 ½ cubit heavy copper ring above the float tank, my personal experience, as well as my clients', has changed, and in some cases, dramatically. I just recently added a second ring above the tank and it seems to have enhanced this overall effect even more. Some of the general comments are that there seems to be a force field, something that holds one and gives added support to the experience. Some have even felt a physical holding of their body. Each person feels this as beneficial and healing. I have had clients report swirling circular lights above them, and a greater sense of expansiveness. Never have I had so many people report "life changing experiences" as since adding the ring. Perhaps it's coincidental that my business has never been as popular as it currently is, and the percentage of clients having such highly positive experiences. At times, it feels as if I'm being plugged into an electric socket of pure bliss, both when I meditate within the ring and float under it. Prior to getting the ring, I was having very difficult experiences of disorientation in the float tank and tremendous fear around these states. These experiences have vanished for me and have been replaced by a deep sense of being embodied and held within a loving field. I want to say thank you so much for making these wonderful tools available. For me, it has been a wonderful facilitator of consciousness expansion.

"Since wearing my Unity Harmonizer, I feel like the frequency of my being has changed and I'm able to function at a much higher level than ever before. I recently took some of the smaller rings and the Acu-Vac Coil to a Mahamudra meditation retreat with me, and found an amazing ease of being able to relax into my awareness such as never before. The sense of relaxation, being held, and greater awareness all seem to go together, and have given me a much higher level of functioning in my life. Each day, my clients share amazing experiences of their floats and how it has affected their lives, and I have a strong sense that much of it is credited to the addition of the ring above the float tank. Thank you so much for bringing these to the world." *S.Z., NY*

RINGS AND HORSES

"I use the rings on our riders and horses all the time. I have one horse that likes a ring on her neck at the shows to calm her, as she is a "Nervous Nellie." I have used the rings on the horses for laminitis, EPM, and colic. And right now, I have a horse experiencing extreme vertigo from EPM and one who suddenly developed Horner syndrome (facial paralysis) that we have hooked up with the rings." *B.H., IL*

SLEEPING WITH THE RINGS

"I have been sleeping with a 3½ Sacred Cubit Ring on the headboard and another 3½ Sacred Cubit Ring on the footboard of my bed. Additionally, I keep a heavy gauge gold plated is la under my pillow with two Plain Jane copper and one 1 Sacred Cubit Rings in Vesica Piscis formation on either side of it. I wear Plain Jane ½ Sacred Cubit Rings on my arms. Suspended over my bed is a personal size gold plated Harmonizer.

"I have been sleeping better, not stirring even once during the night (eight hours average), until I wake up completely clear-headed and refreshed about a half hour before the alarm goes off. Then I take some of the rings to my meditation corner. I've been having unusually lucid dreams. Either I'm a nut case who's taking this too far, or I'm just feeling too darn good to stop myself.

"On an even lighter note, one of the Sacred ½ Cubit Plain Janes I was wearing on my wrist must have slipped off while I was shopping today. In other words, I ended up with a lost Sacred ½ Cubit Ring." *A.C., FL*

A Guest Who Dropped in for Dinner

"Just prior to sitting down to Thanksgiving dinner at a neighbor's house, we heard a loud crash. We thought a car hit the side of their house. We ran out to find a remarkably large goose, the size of a penguin, lying still on its back. I immediately thought of Slim's 3½ Lost Cubit Ring, and ran to get it.

"I held the ring over the goose. He rose up like he was spring-loaded, and I screamed. He flapped his wings three times, lifted into the air, and flew away. I followed his path with the ring until he was out of sight. What baffled us was that the goose was not a Canadian goose. We had never before seen a bird like that." *S.D., NH*

A New Cat Collar

"I have had a great experience with my cat. She had been sick for a long time with various allergies and vomiting. She also had a problem with balance due to an inner ear infection. On my last trip to the vet, the only recourse left was to take her to the vet school for lengthy and costly diagnostic procedures. I put a ½ Sacred Cubit Ring on her, which she wears constantly. She has been wearing it for about four months now and has no apparent symptoms. She is now doing perfectly well, although her hearing is not the best. I'm hopeful that will improve too. A friend, seeing what I did with the ring, put one on her cat. Her cat also has allergies, and is now doing much better. Both cats were not using the litter box, and both have now put that problem behind them." *J.A., WI*

RING EXPERIENCE

"Hardly a day goes by without someone asking us about Slim Spurling's rings, coils, and Harmonizers. All I am able to do is give my experience on this subject. I am not an expert on these devices, but I have been experimenting with them now for many years.

"What I have found is that some of these devices are psychotronic and some are not psychotronic, meaning that they work in harmony with human consciousness. The psychotronic effects explain why some of these devices, such as the Harmonizers work better with some people than others.

"I have found that the Acu-Vac Coil and the rings work simply by their design. They do not seem to rely upon consciousness for their effects. When used for structuring water, the rings do appear to change the quality for the better, not just of water itself, but also of other substances, such as wine and foods. I was in Japan with several expert and professional wine tasters who all agreed the wine that sat in a Slim Spurling ring for a few seconds was dramatically changed. They told me that even cheap wines were changed into fine wines by this process.

"Some of the tasters also were wine sellers, and they purchased big rings in order to run their cases of wine through them, believing they would thereby make a fortune. However, after a few months, they removed the rings because they found that they were beginning to lose money on their expensive wines. Why? Because the people they sold to could tell the difference. Their customers had begun to purchase only the cheap wines. Human nature.

"If for no other reason, these devices are exceptional for learning how energy moves and how it can be changed. I have rings on all the outlets of water in my house because they structure water, and I can taste the difference. It's also important to place them on outlets to your bath or shower. When you take a bath, within twenty minutes, sixteen ounces of water will pass through your skin into the interior of your body. So the water you bathe in is just as important as the water you drink!"
T.N., HI

Rings Help Allergic Reaction to Work Environment

"A 34-year old with complaints of chronic allergic reaction to her work environment was unable to work five days in a row because of headache, sinus congestion, sore throat, burning eyes, etc. She worked alternate days at home (her work is computer based) in order to manage her allergic reactions. The work environment was in recycled air, closed windows, etc. Other office workers reported similar difficulties, but so far nothing had improved or changed. She began wearing a 2 Sacred Cubit Ring around her waist and was relieved of symptoms after a couple of weeks. Two co-workers taped 2 Sacred Cubit Rings under their desk chairs and reported significant decreases in their symptoms, as well. She will wear a 1 Sacred Cubit Ring on a ribbon around her neck instead of the 2 Sacred Cubit Ring around her waist, with the same results. Three of her office mates have purchased their own rings, as they were so impressed with the results. One of them wears it while jogging during allergy season and says it works so well for her, she no longer has to take medicine." *A.A., IL*

Potentized Water Helps Kidneys

"I live in Anchorage, Alaska. I have had several Life-Light Rings for a year and a half. This month, I attended a geostress workshop put on by Merlin Beltain, where I learned some of the uses for the tools. I came home and began to treat our well water (which is excellent) with a ring. I placed a jug of water in the center of a medium ring (1 Sacred Cubit Ring) for 15 minutes. Immediately, I noticed that the water just was easier to swallow and did not upset my stomach. I have a degree of kidney failure and form stones on a regular basis. In addition, I experience a lot of fatigue and other symptoms.

"The things that I want to communicate to you are: 1) In one day I am able to drink more water that is treated in this way; 2) I actually had some detox symptoms -- headache, upset stomach, and increased fatigue for a few days! And, 3) Now I feel good! Much better and my urine is clearing up nicely from its miserable milky grey appearance. I assume that these things are of interest to you, and I will be continuing this treatment. I believe that I will try placing the ring on each kidney area for five to 10 minutes a day and see what happens." *A.B., AK*

WATERING MY YARD

"I would like to relate my experience of watering my yard, using a ring on the faucet. This summer I have used no fertilizers or other soil amendments. I live in a suburban neighborhood and have a deck off the second level which enables me to view several of the neighboring lawns. Mine is by far the richest, darkest green, and most beautiful. Strawberries were planted by the previous owner and they yielded a most delicious crop, despite the fact that while I was away the first two weeks in July, they were barely watered and almost died out. As of today, they are still producing berries. The flower garden is doing exceptionally well. As you can assume, I am on city water. That small ring of Slim's really does wonders. Next year I hope to put in a serious vegetable garden." *F.F., WA*

USING RINGS ON IRRIGATION EQUIPMENT

Using Light-Life rings on irrigation equipment — from the garden hose to the large agriculture pivot irrigation systems — also results in increased biomass. For the garden hose, it can be a ½ Sacred Cubit Ring around your wrist while holding the hose through the ring. Or, place a ring over the sprinkler head. To get the best results, the rings need to be placed at the end of the irrigation system — hose, pipe, etc. — where the water exits. Prior to this, the water is under linear pressure, which confines water from its natural curvilinear flow. The rings change the structure of the water molecules.

HELP FOR A SOLDIER

"I have a report from a high-ranking soldier who broke his hand about 10 days ago. He had heard me in the office talking to another co-worker, and I offered to let him try a 1 Sacred Cubit Ring. He accepted the offer, and slept with the ring each night for two nights. I talked to him after the second night, and he said when he woke up the first morning (the day after the break and the cast was put on); he had no more pain and could move all his fingers. He was amazed. He said he could not do that at all before! On day three, he broke his cast in the palm area and had to have a replacement put on. Upon removing the cast, the medical staff commented that his hand should have been very bruised because he broke all four knuckles. When they removed the cast and looked, very little bruising! Also, the first x-ray after the break showed crooked knuckles where the bones should have been straight. After the second x-ray, the bones were all straight, as they are in a healthy normal hand! Again, the staff was puzzled, "How did this happen?" Ha, ha! I don't think he told them about the ring. He just smiled to himself ....

"Another soldier borrowed my heavy-duty copper 2 Sacred Cubit Ring for back pain he has had for 10+ years. Let me tell you, it was not easy getting it back from him! LOL! He didn't want to part with it, and he is not easily swayed with opinion or just talk. The rings WORK." *R.N., Iraq*

A Healer's Experiences with the Light-Life Rings

"I have been a healer since my near-death experience in 1975 and was guided to work in Arizona where I learned earth healing and house clearing techniques. I use a Tibetan bowl to help identify stressed/blocked/difficult areas. It works for me like a dowsing tool. When an area is clear, it sounds constantly and clearly with many levels of harmonics. When an area is blocked, it stutters and has little clarity and few harmonics. During a recent house clearing, an assistant was trying to sound a bowl in a room, which had very frazzled energies. When we asked the owner, we were told a bi-polar schizophrenic guest has been staying in that room. From the other room, I could hear the difficulty in sounding the bowl, so I walked in with a 1½ Sacred Cubit Ring with three beads, and as soon as I pointed it at the bowl with the intention of clearing the room, the Tibetan bowl sounded clearly (less stuttering and more harmonics). We repeated this experiment in several rooms with the same results. I am so excited about using the rings in the clearings and have started an account to buy a Harmonizer.

"I took the ½ Sacred Cubit Ring and two small Plain Jane Sacred Cubit Rings with me on a trip to assist in some clearings I was guided to do. I used the small rings to place under glasses of water in restaurants. It takes little time to taste the difference in the water. On my birthday, I was offered champagne. I generally do not drink, but when I do take a bit, I try to stick to European and Californian wines because they do not have additives. Other wines give me awful headaches. Being in Europe, I assumed it was European champagne I drank. Later, I started to get the type of headache I get from sulfites/nitrates that generally lasts three days and no OTC pain killer touches. I was distressed, as I did not want to ruin the last days of our vacation. I thought of the ring and put it over my head, wearing it like a necklace. Within five minutes, the headache began to subside. Within 15 minutes it was entirely gone. I am so grateful.

"Recently, I had a client who had an anomaly that doctors called a "hematoma" inside her leg muscle. It felt like one or two soft tumors and different from any I've felt before. I asked her to feel the spot and show me exactly where it was before we started. I placed the 1½ Cubit Ring on the area, and wore two small Sacred Cubit Rings on my arms. I placed my hands on her leg inside the ring, asking for complete healing of her leg if that was for the highest good of all. I saw with inner sight, a large bubble, followed by a smaller bubble, leave her leg. Then I was directed to energetically "close" the area. When I heard that it was done, I removed the ring and asked her to feel for the anomaly. She looked quite surprised when she could not feel it at all. She had already scheduled an MRI this week, and they found nothing." *L.M., AZ*

ANOTHER HEALER'S EXPERIENCE

"We place the small Light-Life Ring inside our ring systems. When people come to the office, I have them stand inside our two 3½ cubit heavy rings (Sacred and Lost), which we have placed one inside the other. Each of these rings has five balls. We had discovered, intuitively, that if you position the balls in five evenly spaced locations, and then offset the balls of the two rings so you basically have 10 balls evenly spaced, the energy is dramatically stronger than any other usage we've been able to come up with." *J.M., Canada*

esoteric, or/and a waste of valuable time. Well, I looked up esoteric in the dictionary. And I quote, "1. Understood or meant for a select few; profound and; recondite. 2. Belonging to the select few. 3. Private; Secret; Confidential. 4. Of Philosophical Doctrine, etc. Intended to be communicated only to the Initiated." Then I looked up recondite. It reads, "1. Hidden from sight; concealed. 2. Incomprehensible to one of ordinary understanding or knowledge: deep. 3. Of relating to, or dealing with something little known or obscure."

"Does this apply or what? I can't thank you enough. The quick and easy return of equilibrium and harmony is a true gift. I believe the Creator intended for you and I to meet."

Dora L. Lofstrom, Ph.D., N.D., D.D., Clinical Researcher, Executive Director of Personal Relations & Board Trustee for The World Natural Health Organization

Everything is energy. Quantum physics has shown us that ultimately everything is light. Science has proven that all energy is interconnected; all life is in communion with and vibrating at levels that reflect the constant evolution toward higher levels of harmony and balance. Chaos is change, the universal ebb and flow, expansion and contraction of this evolutionary process. The Light-Life Tools with their tensor field support and speed up this process. They produce a field of harmony and balance that all in its radius responds to. Given a low and high vibration, the nature of energy is to rise to the higher vibration, its true nature.

All in the harmonious field must rise to the new vibration. This has been demonstrated in the harmonizing of water, the calming of storms, the shift in consciousness. The understanding that all life, all energy is interconnected underscores the power of bringing harmony to one arena knowing it will affect the whole of humanity and life.

What we do here and now is powerful beyond measure. In these times of great chaos, we have been given the tools to offer a higher vibration, a simple and natural solution that works as nature does, simply powerful.

The tools are there to support and accelerate the journey and the events on our life path as we learn to recognize who we are called to be. The tools don't make the choices. They support choices. The tools are not here to live for you. They support you toward being who you are, so remember to always make the highest choices. The tools are based on universal truth and harmony. Always choose the universal truth.

CHAPTER 8
Speed Up Your Healing Process ~ The Acu-Vac Coil

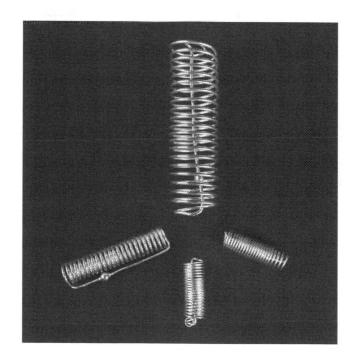

"The Acu-Vac Coil acts like a vacuum cleaner pulling in negative energy on one end, and sending out a beam of positive energy on the other end."

Slim Spurling

BACKGROUND OF THE ACU-VAC COIL

I just finally got tired of making rings one morning. I'd been up since 5 o'clock or so making rings. What else in the world can I do with a piece of wire? So I took a piece of 12-gauge wire, wrapped it on a piece of pipe, soldered the ends together, and tested it. I showed it to a clairvoyant friend. She said, "Oh, the black energy comes in this end and the white energy comes out this end. How fast is it moving?" Well, about how fast you run water through a garden hose. Oh, it's like a vacuum cleaner then – dirty stuff/negative energy in, positive energy out. "Okay, that's all I need to know."

So that evening I had the opportunity to test it on some real pain. The first application was to put the positive end near the pain. It didn't feel bad, but it made the person's head stuffy. Then I just said, reverse it. Change ends. And the energy began to flow out of the body, and the pain disappeared. So that was our first proof, if you want to call it that, or first experience with the coil and the ability to move negative energy from one location and convert to a positive energy so it doesn't foul the environment. But, the original thought I had was what else can I do with a piece of wire? And knowing the polarities of wire, and knowing that you always move in a clock-wise direction, then it was very simple.

RELATING THE CONNECTION OF THE ACU-VAC COIL TO THE CADUCEUS WINDING

The Acu-Vac Coil fit the caduceus definition because the energy field of the loops crosses the energy field of the outside wire at right angles. Or in the case of these coils, the wire comes up the center, but the principle is the caduceus winding. Where the wires cross, the energy fields cross. We're dealing with electromagnetic energy. Every radio wave, every microwave oven running, every television station, every cell phone, every tree, every rock is emitting microwave frequencies at higher and lower energy levels. And when an electromagnetic field encounters a conductor, it moves along the conductor.

Now we have a copper wire, which is a conductor. The energy begins to move, creating what ordinarily would be an electromagnetic field and may actually be electromagnetic in the wire itself. However, it translates into the plane of the ring as a non-electric, non-magnetic field. It's a different form of energy.

Okay, and now we have all of this energy impinging, all this radio energy impinging on the ring or the coil and there's an enormous amount of power running loose in the environment, along with the natural energies. So now we have literally all the power plants in your local area, all of the radio stations, all of the microwave towers, all of the cell phones driving the energy field, but being converted to a positive form of energy.

TECHNICAL INFORMATION REGARDING THE ACU-VAC COIL

The following is a transcript from Mühldorf, Bavaria, Germany (Hotel Bastci), 5/04/2000 Slim Spurling in the company of Katharina Kaffl, regarding the Acu-Vac Coil.

"Every body is surrounded by its own proper atmosphere of this fluid [aether], which grows denser as it recedes from the surface. This is analogous to the atmosphere of excited electricity, which determined bodies once got within the sphere of its attraction to the surface of the electric body. It is to be observed that bodies thus in contact with the excited body remain, some longer, some a shorter time, in contact with that body until they have got an atmosphere of their own. Then they are propelled till meeting with some other matter, at which point they discharge their atmosphere and are attracted and repelled as before." *Cullen*

The above quote by Cullen in relation to aether physics and John Worrell Keely's work may also apply to observations made by myself and Jeanne Dulaney upon the invention in 1992 of the Acu-Vac Coil. Its first application was in the reduction/elimination of pain in Jeanne's neck. Subsequent research applications related to pain were conducted by us and a few thousand (at present writing) students/researchers in many different geographic locations in both the Northern and Southern Hemispheres.

In its simplest description, the Acu-Vac Coil has one end which pulls energy in, and another in which energy flows out. The end closest to the amplifying bead is the outflow, and the end farthest from the bead is the inflow.

In its simplest application, the inflow end is placed on or near the point of pain on the body identified by the person experiencing it. The Acu-Vac Coil is then moved or drawn away from that point at a very slow pace, about one yard or meter per minute. The further the position of the coil from the point of pain, the greater the strength, pull, or inflow to the coil.

This phenomenon of a stronger pull at a distance has been amply and repeatedly reported by many individuals whose pain was pulled out by the coil. Some individuals even report a pull so strong that they tend to lose physical balance – occasionally even requiring bracing against the pull to keep from falling.

With this simple description of the application of the coil to pain as experienced by the human subject, we can leap at once to the known scientifically proven aether physics amply demonstrated by John Worrell Keely, Nikola Tesla, and Wilbert Smith in the late 1800s and early 1900s, and yet only dimly grasped by the advanced physics of the modern sciences of Einsteinian relativity theory and the quantum theory so highly touted by today's scientific academia.

Anyone with an Acu-Vac-Coil in hand properly oriented with the inflow near the pain and outflow in the opposite direction can, if they pay close attention to their own physical sensations or closely observe the subject, experience the reality of aether physics, action at a distance, and the effects of polarity and flow of aether. This reality allows one to stand witness to the natural order, law, and philosophy upon which the aforementioned giants of science built their working hypotheses and operational equipment.

In its first day of existence, the Acu-Vac Coil was submitted to examination by a gifted clairvoyant who stated that negative energy, appearing black or dark grey in color to her vision, was drawn in one end and projected out the other as positive energy, white light to her vision.

That same evening, my wife [at that time] Jeanne returned from the office complaining of a very painful spot on the left side of her neck. We later discovered that the spot coincided with a main acupuncture location on a major meridian most active during that hour (7pm) of the day, hence, during the most optimum time for treatment. After discussing the polarity of the coil with her, she applied the positive-outflow end of the coil to the painful area. In a few moments she said, "It makes my head feel too full." I suggested reversing the coil to draw out the stuffiness, or full feeling, with the negative or inflow end. As this was done, she reported feeling an outflow of energy from the site of the pain, a vacuuming effect, which got stronger as she moved the coil further away. At the end of her reach, she asked me to take the coil and continue moving it slowly further from the pain site.

In a state of complete awe and wonder at what Jeanne was reporting and the apparent miracle I was witnessing, I took the coil and slowly began moving it directly away from her. As I took hold of the coil, I could momentarily see a dark band or cylinder of grey matter, like diesel smoke, emanating from the indicated area of pain and extending outward some four feet to the coil. Above and below this dark energy were two bands of energy, or light, of an unpleasant, yellow-green color. I continued to move away with the coil to a distance of some 20 feet, all the room available in our small apartment. During this time, Jeanne reported a steadily increasing pull and increasing rate of flow of the energy leaving her body.

The sensations she reported moved first down from her neck across the shoulders to her right arm and to the thumb joint which had been broken some years previous. They traveled back up the arm and down the right side to the leg and knee, which had been badly sprained at age 14, then to the foot and an old broken bone in the toe. The sensations continued back up through the leg to the abdominal area, which held the trauma of birthing three children, one by Caesarian, and then later a hysterectomy at age 23. From there, the movement of energy went to a broken rib area near the heart, and then to the head, where she had suffered a concussion from blunt trauma.

This entire process took approximately 45 minutes. At this point, Jeanne's appearance was that of a woman some 30 years younger than her 50 years. She said, "Hold me, and press your hands on my arms, face, sides, hips, legs and feet. Squeeze hard!" After this was done, she wanted to be held and comforted, as she cried and released the emotional charge from all the past trauma and events of both physical and emotional damage.

For the next hour or so, she continued to explore the changes in her physical structure. The joints became so loose and flexible she almost had to learn to walk again. At one point, she shook/shrugged her shoulders, and the entire spinal column spontaneously went into perfect alignment.

The following morning, Jeanne was sitting on the sofa examining her physical structure and noticed that the right leg from the knee to the ankle was curved outward about 1½ inches in relation to the left. Intuitively, she asked me to brace my right hand inside the knee and put firm, steady pressure with my left hand at the point of maximum outward curvature midway between her knee and ankle. I held the pressure, estimated at 25-30 pounds, for about 15 minutes. She then said, "that's enough" and, comparing her legs, found them perfectly straight and aligned.

THE DAY OF RECKONING

In the foregoing narrative, the principle illustrated is that of Cullen's description of the greater density of the aether field at distance from a charged electric body. The key point here is that the pull or action of the Acu-Vac Coil appears to be stronger the further from the body. All life forms are well known to have an aura around them. Sheldrake calls it bio-field or morphic field or aetheric bodies. Those are detectable by dowsing, clairvoyant vision, hypersensitive electro and magnetic instrumentation, ordinary photography, and plain old everyday feel by human neurological response as a sense of touch. This "aura" would then appear to be a kind of electromagnetic field, which is generated by, and radiates from, the elements (C, H, O, Fe, Ca, Mg, Mo, Si, ad infinitum) composing the physical body. This aggregate of atomic elements vibrating/resonating at their individual atomic frequency, compose the solid, liquid, gel, and gaseous structures of matter which hang on some finite, flexible, geometric pattern of energy predetermined by the coding of individual species and the coding of each individual within that species.

I am going to step way out to the end of a new and slender branch of the natural science/natural philosophy tree and propose that the Acu-Vac Coil as discovered and as presently constructed, provides in some as yet indefinite manner, a link between the "aether" matrix of the living body and the overall "aether field" of the planet or even the universal field.

Pain, as we experience it, has analogous phenomena in many areas of study: electrical circuits, auditory harmonics, physical stress in inanimate materials, emotional states, mental states, cultural, social, and environmental areas. Pain can be related to electrical circuitry as an expression of heat in wiring having too much current flowing into too small a wire due to resistance of the wire to too much voltage, i.e., pressure. Localized damage to the wire by stretching, bending, or compression may be the cause of resistance heating. Impurities of lesser conductivity may also cause an increase in resistance, and thus, heating or pain.

The average person will react to disharmonics in musical composition by grimacing in an expression of pain. A well-trained musician may even react violently to disharmonic stresses in a symphonic production. Materials — metals, wood, plastics, glass, and concrete — are weakened or rupture under bending stresses or pain.

In each and every stress/pain area mentioned above, we have witnessed or have reports from students and researchers in the field consisting of the elimination or dramatic reduction of the stress/pain phenomenon in humans, animals, and inanimate objects. Applying the principle embodied in the Acu-Vac Coil relieved mental, emotional, social, cultural, and environmental stress.

Thus, it becomes more and more evident that the Acu-Vac Coil, along with its antecedent and decedent relatives, the Ring, Feedback Loop, and Harmonizer, all exhibit in their applications the same underlying principle. Each tool is known to relieve stress/pain and brings the subject of that stress/pain into balance with the more universal harmonics, or sympathetic vibration.

A few more examples of applications of the Acu-Vac Coil may help the student/researcher to begin to use the tool to reduce stress/pain in his/her personal arena of life. Many of the cited events deal with crisis or emergency situations of extreme stress not too likely to be encountered in daily living, but will serve as an analogy to lesser stresses which can easily be relieved to beneficial effect.

Randy M, one of our early associates and a chiropractic practitioner, uses the Acu-Vac Coil alone to routinely bring about the complete healing and elimination of pain in a broken bone in as little as 10 minutes.

Nancy Z, an equine acupressure teacher, suffered a broken bone in her foot from having it stepped on by a horse she was treating. She placed a ring, an Acu-Vac Coil, and a Feedback Loop in the bottom of a pail of cold water, sitting for an hour with her foot in the water. At the end of this time, there was no pain, no swelling, no discoloration, and no sensation of the broken bone ends grinding one on the other as she put weight on the foot again. She was easily able to stand and work on her feet for the next 12 hours of her scheduled demonstration for a class of students.

Marie, Nancy's co-worker in their business, experienced an abscessed tooth a few months later. Following a thorough dental exam and x-ray confirmation of the abscess on Friday afternoon, she elected to try to save the tooth by alternative therapy methods. Over the weekend various self-treatments with herbs, energy work, heat and cold, etc., had not reduced the pain/infection. Monday morning as she left the farm in route to the dentist's office, she remembered the results that her partner, Nancy, had gotten with the tools. Taking the ring from around a bottle of water on the van's console, she hung it over her left ear, took a mouthful of the "potentized" water, pressed the base of her Personal Harmonizer to the cheek over the painful tooth, and drove about 40 minutes to the dentist's office. Upon arriving at the office, she was experiencing absolutely no pain. She decided to get confirmation from the dentist that the lack of pain was accompanied by some evidence that the condition had abated. Tapping on the tooth with his instrument produced no pain, so the doctor recommended a confirming x-ray exam. The x-ray film showed no evidence of an abscess or abnormality. The doctor was baffled. Marie was delighted, and has retained the tooth to this day with no further complication. This event has been duplicated by several dozen students/ researchers in various countries around the globe over the past several years with the same results.

In the arenas of mental/emotional/social stress, the uses of the tools are illustrated by the following few anecdotes.

One evening in 1995, Jeanne and I were seated in a popular restaurant for dinner. A man and woman arrived and were seated in the next booth. Their relationship was obviously quite strained, as their voices were pitched in loud and angry tones, and their words were derogatory toward each other. Within a few minutes, it appeared they would soon be engaged in a physical battle. Jeanne then took her Acu-Vac Coil from her purse and directed the drawing-in flow end toward the couple, while holding it beneath our table and out of sight. There was an immediate silence between the combative couple in the next booth, which continued for a minute or so as the negative energy between and around them was drawn through the coil. The removal of the negative energy was almost visible and tangible. As it dissipated, the couple burst out laughing, ceased their quarrel, and a half-hour or so later departed hand in hand after a pleasant and agreeable conversation over their supper. Perhaps they could see each other in a different light than in the dark energy fields in which they arrived. Needless to say, Jeanne and I were amazed and very pleased to witness this transformation wrought in such an unexpected manner by the positive influence of the coil.

To further elaborate on the nature of the Acu-Vac Coil and bring the effects *observed into the realms of known, recognized, and duplicable experimental science, I am going to state clearly that the Acu-Vac Coil is a caduceus form of winding; it is and behaves as a super-conductor at ambient temperature; it exhibits an apparently infinite range of frequencies in the electromagnetic spectrum as well as the virtual or scalar spectrum; it will convert a very weak electric voltage input to current or to amperage 400 times greater than the voltage; it exhibits frequencies harmonic to the speed of light.* (ref. Bruce Cathie's grid harmonic mathematics) [Hans Becker's electronic frequency research and discoveries video documentary March/April 2000]

The following data is an interpretation of the video documentation by Slim Spurling, done in Hans Becker's electronics laboratory, April 2000.

With a single wire attached to a ring and a current/ammeter probe attached to an Acu-Vac Coil, Hans demonstrated that the natural frequency of the ring was harmonic with the Acu-Vac Coil and that the coil received the signal from the ring at a distance. The received signal in the coil could be modulated by manipulating the coil with the fingers. By slightly pressing or flexing the coil, deep "Vs" appeared in the oscilloscope graph, indicating several natural energy absorption peaks.

The significance of this absorption of energy by the coil would indicate a probable mechanism by which the coil functions would absorb those frequencies in several octaves of energy from the pain area. The position of the absorption peaks is easily varied by manipulation of the coil and/or varying the input voltage using a musical chord, single note (frequency) as an electrical input, or as an audio input via a precisely recorded electronic frequency converted to audio with a transducer. Simplest of all would be to use the trained human voice, or a tuning fork for the vocally challenged.

Another instance of creating an effect at a distance under measureable conditions occurred sometime in 1995. A very high quality biofeedback machine was attached to the wrist and elbow by stick-on electrodes. The machine's settings were adjusted to zero on the dial to keep a steady tone on the audio indicator. An Acu-Vac Coil was held by another person who approached from a distance of three to four feet. The tone signal faded as the coil was brought within two feet of the arm. The dial tone was brought back to balance, and the coil was moved to within 12 inches of the arm. At that distance, it became nearly impossible to maintain balance and tone on the dial audio. The machine's operation depends on the GSR, galvanic skin response. In electrical terms, that is resistance. To achieve what the coil accomplished in two minutes, a biofeedback subject/trainee would study/ practice for weeks to months.

Apparently, what was witnessed here was "action-at-a-distance." For this to occur, there must be a medium common to both the coil and the flesh between the two electrodes. We will hypothesize that the medium is the aether, so well-known to science in the 1800s, and whose properties were the subject of much experimentation and research by leading natural scientists well into the 1900s. Scorned by academics and funded institutions, a tiny handful of keen observers of nature keep the flame alive. The coil, with its infinite range of frequencies in both the EM and Scalar octaves, with dominant frequency bands harmonic with light, sound, and aether octaves, is able to resonate and entrain the inter-atomic aether matrix of the air space between the coil and the flesh and the atomic substrate of the flesh to bring about a state of lowered resistance or impedance matching between the electrodes. (Ref: Keely, W. Smith, Hans Becker video document)

In electronic or electrical theory and practice, a state of impedance matching between two circuits allows current to flow without hindrance. Hence, the coil with its multiple (essentially infinite) frequencies is able to transmit and induce a state of very low resistance in the skin/flesh between the electrodes.

When a person goes to biofeedback training or therapy, it is to reduce tension/stress, to learn to relax and, in all likelihood, to improve health, whether physical, mental, or emotional. This is done by conscious control of the brainwave states, for example, to impedance match the nerve impulse, thus bringing about a reduction in the GSR (galvanic skin response) or resistance.

In May of 2000 during a trip to South Africa, I had the rare good fortune to meet with Credo Mutwa, an elderly Zulu scholar and medicine man. He is known as a prophet and possessor of ancient tribal knowledge of medicine, culture, history, and the arts. He is skilled in translating the glyphs and signs of written language and symbols inscribed on stone, woodcarvings, and metal objects handed down for hundreds of generations. (See Zecharia Sitchin, "The 12th Planet") I presented him with a coil of my invention, newly produced in 2000. He then expounded at great length on the fact that coils identical to this have been used by the tribal women for various practices in *healing of physical ailments, removal of negative energies from the village, and improving crops. He gave the historical use of the coil in tribal practice as beginning over 4,000 years ago.*

PURPOSE OF THE ACU-VAC COIL

The Acu-Vac Coil acts like a vacuum cleaner in removing negative energy on one end. The other end of the coil projects a positive effect. In its operational function, the coil is designed to employ the fundamental measurements encoded into the Cheops or Great Pyramid of Giza. The basic application of the Acu-Vac Coil, in general, relates more to the physical rather than emotional or spiritual.

DESCRIPTION OF THE ACU-VAC COIL

If you examine the way the Acu-Vac Coil is constructed, it is easy to see that it is just a closed loop. The coils differ from the rings in that there is a one-way energy flow that is selectively directed along the axis of the coil. Coils function like energetic vacuum cleaners. They suck darkness, resistance, and pain through the south end, transmute it, and release it as light out of the north end. The negative energy, or darkness, is converted to positive energy, or light, at the "Bloch Wall." The Bloch Wall is the point where the bead is attached to the coil. When working with this tool, the bead should be away from the person to be healed, so make sure that "the ball is to the wall" whenever you use a coil.

How the Acu-Vac Coil Alters Energy

About two-thirds the distance down the length of the coil from negative to positive, at (or near) the location of the bead, is where the change in energy occurs. For purposes of illustration, this bead is roughly two thirds from the negative input end and closest to the positive output end. This is something we determined very carefully in the production of all our tools - the polarity of the wire and the direction of winding.

Clairvoyants report that as the pain gets sucked out of the body, it appears as if black diesel smoke is moving through the coil. By the time this dark energy exits the north pole of the coil, it looks like pure white light. There is no need for the practitioner to be concerned that what they pull out of their clients will attach to them or contaminate the healing room, because that energy gets transmuted from negative to positive at the bead.

COPPER, GOLD, OR SILVER?

The original Acu-Vac Coils were made of plain copper. Silver-plating and 24K gold plating were added to increase vibratory levels, speed, and smoothness of action. Later, sterling silver coils were determined to be beneficial, as well. As with the rings, many practitioners are of the opinion that the silver plated Large Acu-Vac Coil and sterling silver coils are more conductive and, therefore, superior to 24K gold or copper coils.

ACU-VAC COIL SIZE

Any coil you have on hand will work, so don't let the fact that you only have a small coil to work with prevent you from getting the job done. If you have a choice about which size to use, let common sense and intuition guide your decision. Minor aches and pains experienced by adults, children, and pets respond well to the small Acu-Vac Coil.

LOST CUBIT ACU-VAC COIL

These tools perform well in situations where pain, darkness, resistance, or negativity is rooted at the emotional or mental levels. Lost Cubit Coils seem to suck the truth about the pain out into the open. Once brought to light, the crux of the problem can be addressed consciously and the primary issue is often released instantaneously.

LARGE LOST CUBIT ACU-VAC COIL

Adults, horses, cows, and larger beasts respond better to the large Acu-Vac Coil, as they have more horsepower. We actually made these in response to the veterinary practitioners for use on large animals, but we found that human health practitioners - the healers, the chiropractors - found them very effective. They chose them because of the effectiveness of the time frame. They could get more done in less time, and instead of taking two or three sessions of an hour or two each, they could do it all in fifteen or twenty minutes.

It's been our experience that practitioners find they get very good results. A layperson with little or no experience, and only understanding the principles of the tools, can have a profound effect in maintaining the health and well-being of their family.

The Large Acu-Vac Coil provides a significantly denser tensor field than that found in the ring. These harmonic frequencies appear to correlate with and address the various modal frequencies of the sacred geometric structure of the bio-fields of living organisms. The action of the Acu-Vac Coil would then appear to re-tune or re-align the geometric harmonics.

Sterling Silver Acu-Vac Coil

The sterling silver Acu-Vac Coil has a higher frequency oscillation and a stronger tensor field, which gives it a much quicker action compared to the standard copper 24K gold plated Acu-Vac Coil. Some practitioners report that, in most cases, the action is so rapid that an inexperienced user may not recognize the end point of a session. For an experienced user or practitioner, a 24K gold plated Acu-Vac Coil of the sterling silver variety will greatly shorten the session time in a busy practice.

Using the Acu-Vac Coil

We had access one afternoon to an instrument that was a photon-measuring system, which is basically just a video camera. The output was run through a computer, which could then analyze the quality and quantity of light and show this in graphics. Having access to this in Boulder, Colorado, we had a gentleman with a sore shoulder. He's on camera, and the camera shows a dark shadow on the back of his shoulder.

We just took a coil, and standing 30 feet away from him, actually walked up to him and pulled out this dark shadow, reversed the coil, and put positive *energy back in. Lo and behold, the dark shadow disappeared. It was like we had erased it, and it began to emit light like the rest of the body. So we found that an area of shadow shown by this instrument was equivalent to pain because he had a chronic pain in his shoulder. So, in just a few minutes, there was a major change.*

The further away from the body, the stronger the effect of the coil. And only recently, we discovered that this is related to the higher density of gravity field energy at the perimeter of a galaxy. Okay, so if we assume that our bodies are like a galaxy using the "as above, so below" analogy, then your bio-field has a stronger effect at a distance from the body.

SUMMARY OF PROCEDURAL STEPS

Holding the coil about an inch away from the problematic area and employing a slight circular or in-and-out motion allows the vacuum effect to "couple" onto the pain. This will be felt or sensed by either the client or the practitioner, or both individuals. After the coupling occurs, the coil may start to vibrate, or you may notice that the metal gets hot or cold. Sometimes the person you are working on will tell you that they feel the pain being pulled out.

As soon as any change is registered, either in the person being worked on by the healer, or in the tool itself, keep the coil aimed directly at the trouble spot and slowly move it outward in the auric field, in four to eight-inch increments. The research of Dr. Hartmut Müller has shown that the force of gravity is more powerful at the outer reaches of the galaxies than it is at their centers. Due to the Law of Correspondences, the same is true of the human bio-field. The vacuum effect of the coil increases at a distance, so the further away this tool is held from the body, the stronger the pull will be. In some situations, moving out to distances of twenty feet or more is not uncommon.

THE ACU-VAC COIL USED IN CHAKRA WORK

Chakra clearing is greatly enhanced when performed with a coil. To do this, all you have to do is hold the coil perpendicular to the chakra and wait for change to register in the client, in the practitioner, or as vibration or temperature increase/decrease, in the tool itself. Blockages and shut downs are opened in half the time, with less effort on the part of the healer and the client. Any trauma normally associated with removing these blockages or opening these vital portals in the body is virtually nonexistent. The clearing effects are also much more noticeable and lasting.

APPLICATION OF THE ACU-VAC COIL

The Acu-Vac Coil is not limited to adverse physical conditions. You can use a coil to pull negative energy out of any situation. Aiming the south pole of a coil in the direction of a crying baby, an obnoxious person or group of people, a piece of equipment that isn't working properly, or any set of circumstances that is out of harmony produces positive changes. You can even position a coil in front of a photograph of a sick or troubled person and expect beneficial shifts to occur in a short period of time. Note: A practitioner skilled in remote healing generally uses the photograph as a focal point to concentrate on the individual being healed.

THE ACU-VAC COIL & LIGHT-LIFE RING COMBINATION

A coil can also be used in combination with a ring. The two together augment the effects of both. The light from the ring causes anything that is not of the light to come to the surface, and the sucking action of the coil removes the darkness from the situation or condition immediately. This configuration has proven to be very effective on sprains and broken bones. Any condition that your imagination can come up with to use this "coupling" of tools on will respond very quickly and positively.

ACU-VAC COIL SESSIONS

When you work with a coil, expect the session to last at least fifteen minutes and up to an hour or more.

Katharina Spurling-Kaffl suggests, however, that you trust your intuition. According to some practitioners, it is not uncommon for sessions to take less time now than they used to due to a change in consciousness and the earth's vibration. The tools are adjusting to those changes, and sessions that used to take 20 minutes or more may now only take two to three minutes.

Usually, but not always, a sensation of coolness will appear at the point of pain when the treatment is over. Other signs vary from individual to individual. Some people experience release in the form of expressions of grief or anger or laughter. Others recall past injuries very clearly. It's not uncommon for the client to go into a state of bliss or feel animated and joyful.

Individuals and practitioners should consider whether a rest period after a session is appropriate.

OTHER SUGGESTED USES

The coil is also used to remove "negative" energy from liquids and foods. Water becomes clearer and tastes better. Using a ring and a coil together enhances the benefits of both tools, simultaneously removing "negative" and adding "positive."

The coil may also be held in the hand in the slipstream of an automobile traveling down the highway. With the bead to the rear of the vehicle, the coil appears to clear the air ahead, much like Reich's Cloud Buster. In a similar fashion, a coil laid on the transmission hump in a car seems to result in better mileage, according to one experimenter.

A coil with the drawing or pulling end toward a heat source will remove heat from the source. Painful areas are reported to feel cooler when the pain is gone.

A large coil suspended over crock-pots in my shop prevented the temperature from exceeding 180° for three hours. Normally they would boil in one hour. When the coil was reversed, the pots boiled in about five minutes, with over a 25° temperature rise in that time.

FIELD REPORTS FROM RESEARCH ASSOCIATES

ACU-VAC COIL RELIEVES BEE STING

"I was driving in my car and a bee stung me. I'd had that happen before and usually my face and eyes swell to the point I hardly can see. I have a lot of pain, and this condition usually remains for a few days. This time, I had the coil. So I placed the coil with the bead away from my face right where the sting was. I continued driving home, which took about 45 minutes, and by the time I arrived, I could not even see where the sting was. And of course, no swelling and no pain, nothing like that. I was really very happy. And nobody told me I could do that. This is one of the reasons why I say every household should have at least the coil and the ring in their first aid kit. It's amazing what you can do with them!" *K.S., CO*

ACU-VAC COIL AND 1 SACRED CUBIT RING FOR A BURN

"I went to pour boiling water in my thermos, but missed and poured it over my hand. My hand immediately turned red and was swelling and, of course, painful. I immediately put Traumeel [homeopathic] cream on it and placed a 1 Sacred Cubit Ring around my wrist and an Acu-Vac Coil in my palm. Within 10 minutes, the pain was significantly diminished. Within 1½ hours, I noticed my hand was feeling cold and I felt no burning. I removed the ring and Acu-Vac Coil, and immediately the burning sensation returned. So I replaced them for another 1½ hours. My hand was slightly flushed and sensitive to the touch, like a sunburn, but with no blistering or pain unless I touched it. By the next morning, I had no sensitivity or redness. My host had done the same thing three weeks earlier and still had evidence of blisters." *A.A., IL*

REMOTE HEALING

"From experience, I have found that it is possible to do remote healing with Slim Spurling's tools. I use the sterling silver Acu-Vac Coil and simply hold it over a photo or a digital image on a computer screen of the person to be treated. Just as if you were treating the real person, the coil twitches and vibrates until the work has been completed. This process can take up to an hour, and sometimes one must wait for a few minutes between successive blockage removals. Of course, it is essential to receive a healing request or permission from the person to be treated beforehand." *R.M., Ireland*

TENDONITIS

"I have received gifts from Higher Self, wherein I will buy and have all sorts of products in my cupboard but not use them properly or consistently until someone or some event stirs me to do so. For example, about a week ago, I got tendonitis is my right wrist. So what did I do? I applied the "pomadas" creams and took anti-inflammatory medications immediately, but to no avail. After not sleeping for one night and then again a second night, I got out of bed at 2:30am and decided to use the Acu-Vac Coil. (The Big Daddy-I had never really used it before for anything specific.) Well, it took about 30 seconds to get the pain out of the left part of the wrist and another 40 minutes to get the pain out of the rest of wrist. About 95% of my pain was eliminated at that point. Went to sleep and slept well.

"Next morning I used the Acu-Vac Coil again for five minutes and, bingo, I was clear of the pain and tendonitis. Yesterday, I returned to the office and guess what, Sophia, my secretary had tendonitis in her shoulder. She couldn't lift her right arm, and went and got an x-ray at the health outlet close by. Result - shoulder area swollen. Pain pills prescribed and taken. No reduction in pain or swelling.

"So I got the Big Daddy Acu-Vac Coil and put a small ring around her arm. Had her use the Acu-Vac Coil with my instructions in the office. She was able to lift her arm halfway by the end of the day with only a five to 10 minute application. I told her to keep the ring on during the rest of the day and at night, and also told her to use the Don Croft zapper when she went to bed. When I came into the office this morning at 10:00am, she was jumping with joy. The pain had gone by the time she woke up. She could lift her arm completely.

"She went to the doctor, who took another x-ray. The doctor couldn't believe that there was no swelling or complication in the shoulder/arm area. The x-ray showed that the area was clean. The doctor told her to continue doing what she was doing, but that he found it hard to believe that a piece of spiral copper could do what Sophia claimed that it had done. Fortes Abraços (*Big Hugs*)." *D.N., Brazil*

Driving with the Coil

"I picked up my coil at the CANAM Dowsers Convention in Issaquah, WA, and drove 685 miles back to my home. After reading your book, I realized that I could use it in the car. The next weekend, I drove to San Diego, again a little over 600 miles, this time with remarkable results.

"I have a Toyota Camry with a four cylinder engine. In the last three years, I have never been able to get over 30mpg. On the round-trip to (CANAM), I averaged between 28 to almost 30mpg for over 1300 miles.

"I placed the Acu-Vac Coil on my sun visor aimed at the road ahead and with the bead pointing to the back. I drove on I-5 from Redding to Bakersfield, California, a total of 422 miles, and only used 11.2 gallons of gas. This amounted to a seven mpg increase on flat ground. The round-trip from Bakersfield to San Diego, in the hills with traffic, resulted in 32mpg. I am very impressed! Slim, thank you for the tools." *B.H., CA*

Acu-Vac Coil and Scars

"I'm converted! It's fantastic on scars! I used it on a carpal tunnel surgery scar, one-month post-op. Within minutes, the scar softened and flattened considerably and more so over the next week.

"I used both the ring and the Acu-Vac Coil on a liver tumor removal scar that was one-week post-op. It is already healing with minimal swelling. Prior to using the tools, this young lady said it felt like rocks around the scar, and now it felt lighter and with no rock feeling. I noticed decreased heat around the scar and it was flatter and less red.

"I used the Acu-Vac Coil and ring on a seven-stitch scar on an eyelid three weeks post-op. The injury was a trauma impact cut with bruising and swelling of the frontal orbital bone. I also massaged all around the

area one to two times daily, and it is flattening and becoming less red."
A.A., IL

ACU-VAC COIL AND ACUPRESSURE

"I wanted to share this with you. I do a lot of acupressure and have for some time, so I'm pretty familiar with the process. A couple of months ago, I started using the Acu-Vac Coil on the points instead of acupressure. I have found that the results are more dramatic and longer lasting using the Acu-Vac Coil!

"This is cute, too. My six-year-old daughter had a tummy ache the other night, and she went and got the Acu-Vac Coil. She used it on her tummy and got immediate results. She said, "This works really good! We should thank the man who sent it to us." It was so sweet. It's been great to watch all my kids learning how to use these tools. *They are great teammates in the earth healing process too!" N.S., OR*

ACU-VAC COIL AND A CROOKED FINGER

"One afternoon as my husband and I were talking to a small group about the Light-Life Technology, one woman mentioned how she had injured her middle finger a while ago and since then has not been able to straighten it. It has remained crooked. My husband immediately showed her the Acu-Vac Coil and told her to put her finger inside of it. She laughed and said she didn't think it would do anything, but she did place her finger inside. We continued to talk for a few minutes longer, and then she pulled her finger out of the coil. To all of our amazement, it had straightened out." *S.A., PA*

MY MOTHER'S EXPERIENCES WITH THE ACU-VAC COIL

"I placed an Acu-Vac Coil on the side table by my mom's chair. At first she noticed a slight pain in her hips, then a slight sensation of pain going up her lower spine. She has a damaged disk in her lower back, but her hips are OK, I think. She didn't at first notice the Acu-Vac Coil, and wondered what that slight sensation was. Then she saw the coil and told me how she felt. Now she has the Acu-Vac Coil on her bedside table and claims that her back is feeling better." *S.Q., CA*

ACU-VAC COIL AND MY FAMILY

"The first time I used the Acu-Vac Coil (I bought the large one) was absolutely amazing. I used it on my husband and my two sons. My husband has been ill for several years and, in fact, has not worked since February of this year. He has severe arthritis and very difficult to control diabetes, amongst other things, although those seem to be the biggies. We came across a product that has been very effective to detox the body, and the morning of the Acu-Vac Coil treatment, he was on his second big detox in two months (most of which seemed to be from the lungs at the time). I began to work on whatever area he felt he needed to have done. He closed his eyes and would tell me where he felt energy work going on. It wasn't always where I was pointing that he was feeling it - interesting how some things began to tie together. The coil would change temperature, and when I began to work on the lungs, the coil became very, very heavy. In fact, my arms were sore the next day from the weight! Before the treatment, he had a cough that was the beginning of another icky detox (the first detox took an entire month of very severe coughing). There was a major odor in the room in the morning, as well. Let me tell you that AFTER the treatment, his cough was almost over! As with most arthritic people, he loves a hot bath to soothe the joints. But he realized that he could only stand the water about half as hot as usual. And in the morning there was NO detox odor at all! For some time after this, his blood sugars even stabilized.

"I also worked on my sons, ages 12 and 13, who are at that wonderful hormonal age and seem to sometimes pick on each other in the mornings. "I don't want to eat with him!" "He's smacking!" You know the routine. Anyway, the very next morning after I had worked on them, they sat peacefully at the table next to each other, happily eating, and one was even reading a book! My 18-year old son came into the kitchen and I elbowed him and pointed at his two brothers. He looked at them and then asked, "How much did that cost?"

"My husband says I snore, so that same evening after I'd worked on everyone else, I worked on myself. I've done energy balancing for the last couple years on others, so this was a treat to be able to work on myself! My husband told me the next morning that he could barely hear me breathe all night I was so quiet. I believe that having done energy work for the last couple years has allowed me to 'feel' what the coil is doing, and it's amazing! I really love it! What an awesome tool!" *J.C., VA*

THE ACU-VAC COIL AND PAIN RELIEF

"I used the large gold plated Acu-Vac Coil on a friend with an advanced case of cancer which had metastasized throughout her body. The friend was taking morphine medication orally every three hours for temporary pain relief. The Acu-Vac Coil provided pain relief within a few seconds of its application when used in the area of the head, back, internal organs, and various bones.

"The placement of a gold plated copper 1 Cubit Ring on top of the head also provided quick pain relief not only for the head area, but for the entire upper body (since the spinal column is aligned with and below the ring when the person was sitting).

"In a situation where the same person's lungs were partially filled with fluid, the application of this device resulted in the expulsion of a substantial amount of fluid through coughing. This eliminated the need to go to the hospital emergency room to have the fluid removed by insertion of a large needle through the back.

"The Acu-Vac Coil was used on the lungs in the following way: The device was held about three inches away from the body with the capacitor ball furthest from the body. After about 30 seconds, the direction of the device was reversed, with the capacitor ball closest to the body. This was done for each lung, one at a time. Coughing up of fluid occurred in less than four minutes. The optimal procedure was determined by dowsing and reconfirmed by a positive response from the recipient of the treatment.

"The preliminary indications are that the large Acu-Vac Coil and the gold plated copper rings can be valuable tools in providing quick and natural pain relief for people suffering from chronic pain. I hope that my experience will encourage others to experiment with these products." *S.Q., CA*

Pleasant Dreams with an Acu-Vac Coil

"I'd like to share some interesting stories about my experience with the Acu-Vac Coil. Slim created this short-circuit, gold plated copper coil because at one end it produces a sort of suction, while on the other side, energy emerges. It, therefore, produces a vortex field of subtle energies which one can experience when placed under one's pillow during sleep. Dreams become much more vivid! It is truly amazing, as it seems to stimulate the pineal gland. I brought my Acu-Vac Coil on my yearly visit to Germany and showed it to one of my old high school friends. I left it with him and his wife so they could try it out. First, his wife used it for one night and she felt like she was inside a cocoon, a very nice and pleasant feeling, and had a perfect night's sleep. My friend had the same experience when he tried it out the next night. Then they gave it to their youngest son, and he slept so wonderfully that he did not want to return it! I let him have it. Months later I asked my friend if his son was still using the Acu-Vac Coil, which he confirmed, adding that only once in a while were he and his wife allowed to 'borrow' it!" *S.F., NV*

CHAPTER 9
Eliminate Disruptive Energies ~
The Feedback Loop

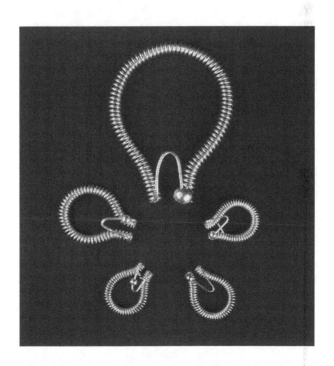

*"In using the Feedback Loop, you're energetically at a higher level,
perhaps even higher frequencies. So it's a very
powerful tool."*

Slim Spurling

BACKGROUND OF THE FEEDBACK LOOP

The Feedback Loop came as a result of Bill Reid studying Tom Bearden's work on phase conjugation. Bill said to Slim, "We've got the Acu-Vac Coil now; it should be easy to make another tool to incorporate Tom Bearden's findings." Slim sat down at his work bench, and the Feedback Loop was born.

PURPOSE OF THE FEEDBACK LOOP

The Feedback Loops pull out negative energy and immediately put back positive energy.

Bill Reid describes it as follows: "The idea is to take the negative energy from an injured part of the body, mirror that energy, change the phase, and feed it back into the body. This process is called a wave canceller."

STANDARD SACRED CUBIT FEEDBACK LOOP

Here's what a trusted clairvoyant had to say about the Standard Sacred Cubit Feedback Loop: "Now let's talk about what energies are being transformed into the body. The Sacred Cubit Feedback Loop works just like the larger one, although in a gentler manner. When you position it facing you, it draws higher energies into your body. Place the Feedback Loop in a vertical position next to your bed on a nightstand, for example, when you go to sleep. It stops disharmonious energies and microwave energies from invading your environment. Positive energies flow in like a stream."

BIRTH OF THE MAGNUM FEEDBACK LOOP

Katharina Spurling-Kaffl was approached by a customer with a request for an additional ring on the Sacred Cubit Feedback Loop, just like on the sterling silver Feedback Loop. She asked her shop craftsmen to add two little rings so as not to confuse it with a 24K gold plated sterling silver FBL.

CHAPTER 9

SACRED CUBIT FEEDBACK LOOPS WITH TWO RINGS — PERFECTION!

"Some weeks ago I ordered two more standard Feedback Loops. I asked that time to see if the company would add a ring onto them, similar to the one on the Sterling Silver FBL that I purchased previously. The standard Feedback Loops arrived with TWO rings attached to each one. The minute I saw them, it was obvious that the two rings were perfect and when I held one in my hand, I couldn't even imagine it with only one.

"Intuitively, for what it's worth, I knew the power had been considerably increased from the original FBL. In addition, I got that the Golden Ray was added along with other attributes. I had to look up what the Golden Ray is referred to, as I was not familiar with its characteristics. I understand that its presence has become more prevalent on the planet in recent months. As to the other attributes, this tool needs to be used by someone who has been using the original FBL on a regular basis. I'm not easily impressed, but this little tool gave me the impression that what I've seen or experienced isn't anything compared to what it can ultimately do. The two rings created a different level of power and dimensional capabilities. The two Feedback Loops each have their place and uses, and one does not replace the other.

"I asked a friend, a well-respected and successful acupuncture practitioner, to use the tool. She had it for one week and of course used it judiciously, as her clients are not accustomed to other 'tools' being used. She used it on herself first while I was there and was amazed that in less than two minutes her toes, which she had been unable to move for over a year, were moving freely. I left it with her.

"I feel compelled to mention that the silver FBL made it abundantly clear that she is perfect as she is; there are no additional 'levels' that are not already contained within her and to not even think of additional loops!!!"
Anonymous

Large Lost Cubit Feedback Loop & the Small Lost Cubit Feedback Loop

A superb healing tool, the Lost Cubit Feedback Loop pulls out any energy that is blocking the resistance of perfect health. If there is an imbalance in the body, position the Lost Cubit Feedback Loop there; if you are unsure of any imbalance, try placing it on the solar plexus, as this affects the whole body.

Stand the large Lost Cubit Feedback Loop up by making a little holder for it. It then becomes an excellent tool to help with balancing the electromagnetic fields within in an office or house. In a vertical position, the large Lost Cubit Feedback Loop blocks harmful energies. Position the Lost Cubit Feedback Loop towards you for two to three minutes, and it will clean out the solar plexus. When you flip it upside down, you pull in energy from the crown chakra. There is a stronger outward effect when the bead is upside down. A Lost Cubit Feedback Loop brings you into higher emotions and transfers calmness into the emotion when held in the heart area. This tool is ideal in the realm of physical issues, too. Let's say a person has back issues and wishes to pull out what is causing the pain. A friend or practitioner holding the Lost Cubit Feedback Loop against the intruding pain for two to three minutes puts remembrance of healing back into the body. This is accomplished by pulling from the crown chakra in the person's back where the pain initiated.

The small Lost Cubit Feedback Loop works on the same principle as the larger Feedback Loop. Hold it with the bead facing you as you are sitting, and it will speak to the energies in the room. When the bead is facing away from you, it is pushing away what is not in harmony and feeds to you what is in harmony.

New Dimension Lost Cubit Feedback Loop

The New Dimension Feedback Loops work differently than either the Sacred or Lost Cubit Feedback Loops and have some intriguing uses. When an individual is working with a New Dimension Lost Cubit Feedback Loop, they should point it with the round side towards their body so that the bead is on top. It removes mental, emotional, spiritual, physical, and even karmic, blockages. Many people hold it at their solar plexus to reverse external energies coming in that are creating blockages. Meditate for two to four minutes as this Feedback Loop goes through every chakra, clearing and transferring blockages. It is important to remember to breathe! Imagine little doorways at the end of your head opening up to let out excess energies. As it moves through the body and all chakras are balanced, face the New Dimension Lost Cubit Feedback Loop towards you and it will put harmonizing energy back into your system. People who have been going through chemotherapy may find this tool especially helpful.

The New Dimension Lost Cubit Feedback Loop is comparable with a magnet. It balances out your energy field, your chakras, and your matrix. This harmonizing balance occurs in the physical, mental, emotional, and energetic realms.

DESCRIPTION OF THE FEEDBACK LOOP

The Feedback Loop is just a narrower coil, a smaller diameter coil, and we found that the energy flowing through the Feedback Loop is a higher velocity. If this standard sized coil has a flow like a garden hose, then this Feedback Loop would be more like a high pressure car wash - a narrower beam, and it would draw energy from, say, a point here in my hand, and feed it back directly into that point. That's what we call phase conjugate mirroring. So we're pulling out energy at a certain frequency and then returning that same energy at 180 degrees out of phase. What this does is cancel the original frequency. So it goes to zero. If you have a frequency causing pain, this would cancel that frequency at the source and consequently eliminate the pain. So it's just a different version of the coil and can be used as a stand-alone, or it can be used in combination with the Acu-Vac Coil and/or the rings.

The Feedback Loops are created in three sizes: Standard Sacred Cubit, Standard Lost Cubit, and Large Lost Cubit. The materials used are copper, 24K gold plating, silver plating, and sterling silver.

- *Standard Sacred Cubit Feedback Loop:* copper that is 24K gold plated, sterling silver, and upon request – silver plated
- *Standard Lost Cubit Feedback Loop:* copper that is 24K gold plated, and upon request – silver plated

- *Large Lost Cubit Feedback Loop:* silver plated and 24K gold plated

APPLICATION OF THE FEEDBACK LOOP

One of our practices when we're using the coil is to pull the negative energy out, reverse the coil, then put the positive energy right straight back into the person. Reversing the coil to return the positive energy isn't necessary with the Feedback Loop because everything is happening simultaneously. In using the Feedback Loop, you're energetically at a higher level, perhaps even higher frequencies; so, it's a very powerful tool.

How to Use the Feedback Loop with the Acu-Vac Coil

When addressing a point of pain – or more particularly, a generalized area of pain as is commonly found across the shoulders or across the top of the pelvis – the loop may be used in conjunction with the coil to aid in breaking up the electronic ridge usually associated with the pain.

- *Hold the Feedback Loop in one hand, the Acu-Vac Coil in the other, and slowly sweep across the pain area.*
- *Start close to the body and gradually, over a period of 10 to 15 minutes, increase the distance of the tools from the body - up to 15 to 20 feet.*
- *There are no formulas or rituals connected with this process. The exact mechanics can be improvised according to what feels right to the user and subject. Verbal communication between the two is therefore encouraged, but not absolutely vital for success.*
- *The devices may be used solo by placing them on an even surface at pain level and slowly walking/inching away, or by moving the body to relocate the affected point.*

There is a tremendous degree of freedom to operate the devices. Do what works, follow intuition, and observe self/subject closely to see and sense what is happening. Let the subject tell you what needs to be done.

WATER TREATMENT USING THE FEEDBACK LOOP AND COIL CONFIGURATION

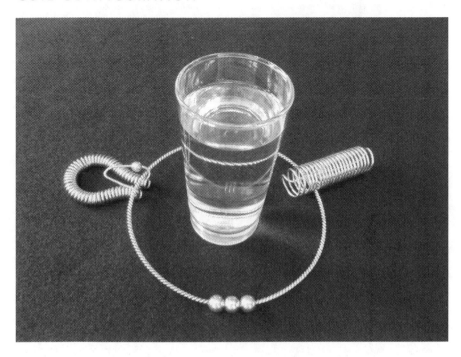

One of the early combinations we used was for potentizing water using a coil hooked onto a Feedback Loop. The Feedback Loop was then hooked into a 24K gold plated ring. This combination drew out the negative energy from a container of water. What we found, by radionics testing and by direct experience, was that if we place water in a configuration like this for a period of twelve hours, the potency or the vitality - the energy quantity in the water - goes off the radionics scale, goes clear off the scale. On experimental application - in other words, just drinking nothing but that water for the next week - you'll find that your requirement for food will go down, your energy level will go up, and your requirement for sleep will be reduced considerably. So, these are effects that we observed both personally and through the reports of many, many other people. We call this the super-potentizing configuration.

The overall potency, or the number of atoms affected, increases over time. And if you leave the jug sitting there and refill it periodically, it's always ready. The texture of the water changes. It's softer, milder, and there's a completely different flavor. And usually within a few minutes to a half hour on a large quantity of water, the chlorine odor completely disappears. I can't say if that's normal or natural, but certainly you can't taste or smell any odors coming from water that's set in a ring for a short time. Ice even melts faster.

EXPERIMENTING WITH WATER

Below, Slim describes an experiment testing two bottles of water. The first bottle is not treated with any Light-Life Tools. The second bottle has an Acu-Vac Coil placed beside it.

This bottle was treated electrically, but did not have a ring or a coil in its proximity. Now, the other bottle, where we can see the beam, developed a very strong colloidal content of particles. The waters are identical, having come from the same source. They've been treated identically, except for the fact that a coil is being introduced into the vicinity of the cloudier bottle. Colloids are known to be the most absorbable of mineral sources, and so any mineral that was dissolved in this water is more available as a colloid than it would have been in a solution or ionic state. This is a brand new discovery in science. There's just nothing we know of that's ever been reported like this.

FIELD REPORTS FROM RESEARCH ASSOCIATES

GIANT ACU-VAC COIL AND FEEDBACK LOOP: DIVERTICULITIS

"I was in Brazil this summer after being away for a year and a half. I found my grandmother very ill and in bed when I arrived. She has been suffering from diverticulitis for the past three years. The doctors have not been able to reduce her pain or have any kind of success in her treatment, not even through her strict diet.

"She was lying there in bed with so much pain on the left side of her abdomen that I could barely touch her skin without her moaning. I could feel that side, as hard as a rock and very swollen.

"She asked me to help her in any way, so I offered to use my tools. I was guided to use the giant Acu-Vac Coil. While I was "vacuuming" her pain, the tool was vibrating tremendously even while distancing from her body. I could feel how congested her intestines and her abdominal area were. After filling the area with light using the positive side of the Acu-Vac Coil, I whispered words of love and compassion to her. I then used the Feedback Loop throughout her abdominal area and intestines, still holding the vibration of love in my heart. I tried to finish the session with Reiki, but still, I could not touch that area at all. I left feeling a little sad and frustrated, for I thought whatever I had done still wasn't enough to relieve her from that terrible pain. The next morning, before 8am, my grandmother called. She normally doesn't get up before 11am I thought, I hope she's OK. She was so excited to tell me that she was without pain. So much joy came through her words as she said, "It was as if you had reached inside of me and pulled the pain out with your hands! When can you come again?!!" I told her that I would see her in three days. I couldn't believe my eyes when I arrived that day. She was walking around and in no pain. When she laid down and I touched her belly, I could massage it deeply and strongly. Her abdomen and her left side were very soft and not at all swollen! She then turned around and asked me to do her right side. I asked her if it was still hurting. She answered, "No, no, it's not hurting, but just in case it should hurt some day." Before I left, she had me write down the name of the tool, the Acu-Vac Coil, and the words Quantum Physics, so she could explain to the doctor what had happened!" *T.R., Brazil*

HELP FOR ACHING HEELS AFTER A LONG DAY

"A middle-aged friend was unable to lift her heels off the ground while walking. This occurred as a result of changing her work-out routine and doing six consecutive hours of chair massage at a fitness center. I asked her to give me one minute with the small gold plated Feedback Loop. I ran it up and down the backs of her legs (at about a five to twelve inch distance) from her knees to the Achilles tendons. I asked her if it had helped, and at first she was doubtful. Then she walked around my living room with a completely normal gait, lifting her heels without pain or stiffness. One minute was all it took. I have also noticed that the tools do not need to be energetically cleaned as often as the crystals I use in healing. They seem to have a self-cleansing property." *A.C., FL*

CHAPTER 10
Clean Air and Water without Chemicals ~ The Harmonizer Family

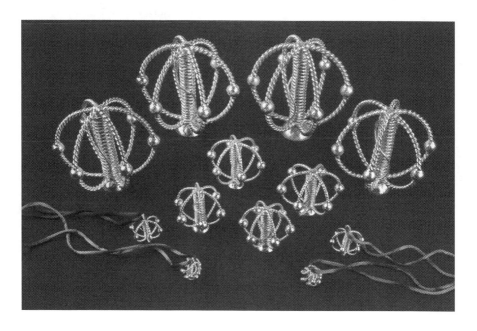

*"I believe the Harmonizer technology can
re-harmonize human nature."*

Slim Spurling

BACKGROUND OF THE HARMONIZERS

You'll find this chapter organized a little differently due to the extensiveness of the material. Each Harmonizer will be discussed, followed with relevant field reports.

The Harmonizer is a combination of rings and coils. I'd like to describe how we came to do this. We first started by spinning a ring in a vertical position, and we found that created a somewhat unpleasant energy field. And it didn't feel good to many of the sensitives. So we thought, well, what happens if we put two rings together? Now we have an energy beam coming out both sides of the 24K gold ring and an energy beam coming out both sides of the copper ring. This creates an effect like a cylinder or a flashlight beam. When we intersected a third ring, all of a sudden the clairvoyants were telling us that we had a spherical field – more like a donut-shaped field. And it didn't appear to have much, if any, motion to it. It was suggested that we put a coil in the center.

Well now we have motion in the energy field, in this toroidal or donut-shaped energy field, so that positive energy is coming out through the top of the field, coming back around, sweeping through, pulling all the negative energy from the environment into the base of the Harmonizer through the coil, and transmuting it again to a positive energy out the top in this donut-shaped, toroidal field. What we're able to do with the coil placed in the center is to create a motion of flow. This is now three-dimensional instead of two-dimensional in the form of a cross. So that was a major discovery.

The Harmonizer emits a cosmic light field or L-field and has a positive output. To the clairvoyant, it appears to emit a coherent holographic light field. It is an "active" tool, in that subtle energies are continually in motion in the large light energy field around it. An individual's own energies are set into motion too, continuing as long as one is in its presence! The Harmonizer can be closed down by placing it in a ring. The energy is then contained in the new cylindrical column and the ring will send it on an upward path.

DISCOVERY - AMPLIFYING THE ENERGY FIELD

Exactly what do we have here? We started with a small Harmonizer, the one we call the Environmental Harmonizer, roughly the size of a golf ball. And at rest, just sitting on the table with no acoustic drive - and by acoustic drive I mean simply placing earphones on either side of the harmonizer - the energy field is approximately a 100-foot radius. It's a limited field. It doesn't get any bigger than that, or not much bigger until you add the sound. The minute you add the sound, the energy field goes from a 100-foot radius out to a 15-mile radius. So we're affecting a really huge area of atmosphere, soil, and water. Our first experiments showed us that with the frequencies of the water molecule being played into the Harmonizer with the earphones, the acoustic drive expands that energy field out tremendously.

Our firsthand observation was that the air smelled fresh. This was during a time in Denver when the brown cloud was in national headlines. Since we could smell the air freshening up, we now had an acoustic air cleaner using this energy field.

PURPOSE OF THE HARMONIZERS

The various Harmonizers are for personal, environmental, and agricultural applications. There's quite a demand for these, and that's been developed because of their unique properties in being able to clean up atmospheric air pollution. And that can extend right on down to the Personal Harmonizer, which is a very small unit, not much bigger than the ball of my thumb. This is used to keep your personal atmosphere strong and healthy, and that's your bio-field, your aura.

The first Harmonizers were very small devices and were designed to reduce electromagnetic interference in the home, to help clean the air in the house, and to improve the outside environment right through the walls. Your local environment – your neighborhood or even a small town – would reap the benefits of one individual having this tool in their home. We went then to the larger ½ Sacred Cubit size of Agricultural Harmonizer, as this was designed to handle large scale ranching and farming operations. It has also been used very successfully in clearing air pollution over sizeable areas up to a 65-mile radius. We have Agricultural Harmonizers distributed almost worldwide on all continents, and they're in daily use by individuals. And we have hundreds and hundreds of reports of the environmental benefits that occur: more wildlife, better plant growth, greater crop yields, and a much more peaceful environment.

Note: Slim referred to the Sacred Cubit Harmonizers exclusively in this last passage as they were the only Harmonizers available at the time of this lecture.

Please be aware that the range of the Harmonizers today may not extend out as far as previously stated because of increased pollution and density of EMF.

DESCRIPTION OF THE HARMONIZERS

SACRED CUBIT AND LOST CUBIT ENVIRONMENTAL HARMONIZERS

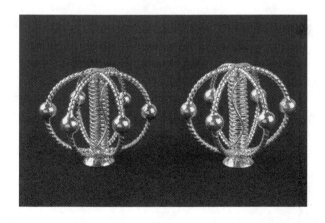

The Environmental Harmonizer may be used in clearing earth energies and creating a more harmonious atmosphere. Farm fields flourish in its environment. Plants grow lush, full, and strong. Birds, butterflies, and worms thrive, and all life forms in the area prosper as they receive its beneficial energy. It is an "active" tool, in that subtle energies are continually in motion in the large light-energy field around it. An individual's own energies are set into motion too – continuing so long as you are in its presence! The field diameter of the Sacred Cubit Environmental Harmonizer is about a 100-foot radius, or 15 miles when activated with the Environmental Clearing CD. It measures 2" x 2." The Lost Cubit Environmental Harmonizer's field diameter is also a 100-foot radius, but increases to 25 miles when activated with Environmental Clearing CD. This Harmonizer measures 2.5" x 2.5."

All Environmental Harmonizers are constructed from copper, then either:

- *plated with eight alternating layers of silver and 24K gold, starting with silver and ending with 24K gold*

OR

- *plated with nine alternating layers of silver and 24K gold, starting with silver and ending with silver.*

Denver Pollution Clearing Experiment

We decided to do another experiment. We placed one of the Harmonizers in front of the boom box speakers, turned on the tape, and within a few minutes my acquaintance said that he could "feel" the energy field expanding through him. Soon, the air smelled like ozone again. Since we had a lot of air pollution in Denver at that time, I wanted to see if we could create this freshening of the air effect over a larger area.

We made copies of the tape and distributed them to ten people in the area who each had one of my Environmental Harmonizers. At 1pm on March 18, 1994, our group was scattered on a line from Colorado Springs to Fort Collins. That is a distance of 140 miles. We had several units in Denver, one in Boulder, one in Fort Collins, and so on. It was a pleasant day with a few scattered clouds and a slight breeze. Once we turned the tapes on, within a few minutes we got a kind of hazy moisture in the air. Previously, it had been quite clear. We played the tapes for one hour. By 7pm, there was not a sign of air pollution whatsoever. It was so clear you could see a candle flame 60 miles away on the horizon. Looking out across the flat valley up to the plains where they rise to a greater height than the city, I was absolutely blown away. I pulled over on the side of the road and cried for joy for an hour. Just to know that finally there was a solution to this terrible condition that almost all cities were experiencing. I never saw L.A., but Denver was the big news item. Since then, we have introduced this technology around the globe through the efforts of private individuals. They've seen their environment improve dramatically in every case. A lot of people noticed. At noon the next day it was so incredibly clear that the weatherman on Channel 4 said, "Folks, you can see Utah today." We have operated with different tapes and frequencies and different size Harmonizers continuously in Denver for the last three years (1994-1997). [There are still many Harmonizers operating in this area as of 2012.]

INCREASED MARINE LIFE

In Provincetown, in the Cape Cod area (in 1996), one of our associates had been playing the Harmonizer with the Environmental Clearing tapes and also using the Light-Life Rings. She reported that they had the best whale and dolphin watching, clearer water, more seaweed, and a greater number and variety of fish than the local fishermen had ever seen in the area. There may be an application here in cleaning offshore waters. Hopefully, we can begin to clean up lakes and rivers with this technology.

HOW THE HARMONIZER EFFECTS POLLUTION

I wish I had all of the chemistry. One thing we do know is that carbon monoxide disappears first. Let's say in a city environment at rush hour we can watch the carbon monoxide levels drop from multiple digits up in the 70, 80, 100 range down to single digits. We've seen this occur within an hour and over a huge area – like LA County! We've got the air pollution readings, and the prediction is it's going higher. It doesn't. With multiple units operating 24/7, it absolutely drops down to single digits. And this, with only the little Environmental Harmonizers.

FIELD REPORTS FROM RESEARCH ASSOCIATES

CRUISING WITH A HARMONIZER

"In early September of 2011, my beau and I flew to Seattle and then boarded the MS Oosterdam, a Dutch cruise liner, bound to southeast Alaska. Almost nothing could mar my excitement of finally getting to see what is known as "the last frontier." Almost nothing, that is, except for cold, wet, rainy weather which is what was predicted for the entire seven days we were on board. Fortunately, I had a gold plated Sacred Cubit Environmental Harmonizer tucked into my luggage. We set up the Harmonizer in our stateroom and activated it using the CD. We weren't practiced in the use of the Light-Life Tools, but I had been instructed to direct my intentions to the Harmonizer. Michael and I both desired weather that would allow us to enjoy our excursions at the various ports we would be stopping at. We each silently spoke those intentions, hoping to see good results. To our delight, it rained only slightly before we disembarked in Juneau, our first stop, and then the sun came out! We enjoyed a stunning canoe trip around Mendenhall Glacier in seasonably comfortable weather. Back onboard, we overheard crewmembers saying, "We haven't had a day this beautiful in weeks." Hmm, maybe our Harmonizer was responsible for this glorious day, we thought. Indeed, the weather the next six days was as unexpected as the first day. We continually heard crew and passengers giving thanks for the surprisingly good, clear weather. Our adventure ended too quickly, but with the knowledge that the Harmonizer helped create a most memorable cruise experience and exploration of our 49th state for the 2200 passengers on board the MS Oosterdam." *D.C., CO*

RED TIDE MITIGATION PROJECT, TAMPA BAY AREA

"The Red Tide is a nasty algae that kills marine life and generates a toxic aerosol that is a health hazard to humans. It has cost the state of Florida millions in lost revenue in resort areas and fisheries. In recent years, these toxic blooms have become more chronic and severe. A bloom started last January and has never fully dissipated. The purpose of this project is to mitigate the health hazards created by pollution in area waterways, through the use of methods inspired by higher consciousness.

"The Environmental Harmonizer was sound activated for two hours at Siesta Beach. The observations, based on several reports, indicated that it was the first weekend this year that there had been no trace of Red Tide at Siesta Key.

"Note the front page headline in the <u>Sarasota Herald Tribune</u>:

RED TIDE TAKES A BREATHER: THE AIR IS CLEAR, THE FISH ARE ALIVE AND NO ONE KNOWS WHY

"And, a secondary main article, front page:

TOURISM OFFICIALS HEAVE A SIGH OF RELIEF AND WOULD PREFER NOT TO TALK ABOUT IT

"This is the first time in 10 months that Red Tide has abated in the area. Scientists are baffled because none of the measurable indicators or factors they know can account for its sudden disappearance. The Storm Chaser, Environmental, and Agricultural Harmonizers were all sound activated 24/7 since October 21, 2005. They were placed on a radionics map of the Gulf of Mexico and surrounding landmasses. The successful use of the Harmonizers in the Tampa Bay Area is reminiscent of the success in the 1998 Red Tide Reduction Experiment in the San Diego Bay Area." *A.C., FL*

ENVIRONMENTAL HARMONIZER HELPS WITH A BITTER ATTITUDE

"I purchased an Environmental Harmonizer in August, 2000, with the idea of clearing out the air around here. It is mostly agricultural dust. I play the Environmental Clearing CD twice a day, around sunrise and sunset for an hour and a half usually. The air is somewhat clearer, but not as dramatic as I had hoped for. There has been an unexpected side effect, though.

"My ex-wife lives close by, near enough to be inside the Harmonizer's field without musical excitation. About ten weeks after using the Harmonizer, her attitude toward me has changed from bitter enmity to friendly, pleasant, and co-operative. The negative energy coming from her house toward mine was so strong that I had to put up Feng Shui mirrors to reflect it. This was long before I ever had any of Slim's products. I took the mirrors down over the last weekend. And no, we will not get back together. Our lives have taken different directions, but at least the fierce hate is gone. This is good for her soul and mine, too. My psychic friend tells me that she won't carry any unresolved anger with her when she leaves this earth, meaning that we two won't have to work it out in some other life. Slim, you are wonderful!!" *F.F., WA*

SACRED CUBIT AND LOST CUBIT AGRICULTURAL HARMONIZERS

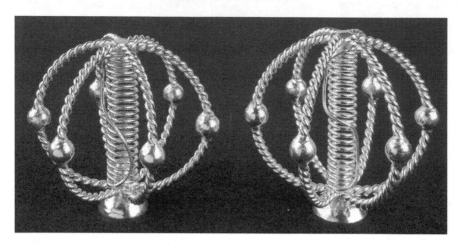

The working field diameter of both the Sacred Cubit and Lost Cubit Agricultural Harmonizers is about a 1½-mile radius. Their applications are the same as for the Environmental Harmonizer, but with a wider range when activated with the Environmental Clearing CD. The Sacred Cubit Agricultural Harmonizer's effective radius then increases to 65 miles, and the Lost Cubit Agricultural Harmonizer's effective radius reaches to approximately 85 miles. The size of the Sacred Cubit Agricultural Harmonizer is 4" tall x 3.5" wide. The Lost Cubit Agricultural Harmonizer is 4.5" tall x 4.5" wide.

The difference between the Sacred Cubit and Lost Cubit Harmonizers is the direction of the movement of energies. According to the latest information Katharina received from a clairvoyant reading, while both measurements work on both areas, the Sacred Cubit seems to have more of a vertical energy and is best used for cleaning the air. The Lost Cubit seems to have more of a horizontal energy and is best used for soil and water applications. Reports point to increased and rapid plant growth and indicate the Lost Cubit Harmonizer is perfect for cleaning water of all kinds of pollution. To a certain degree, both harmonize the environment and the person in the environment, but the movement of energy is different.

APPLICATION OF SOUND TO INCREASE FIELD RANGE OF HARMONIZING ACTION

At rest, the field radius on the Agricultural Harmonizer is about a mile and a quarter. With the acoustic addition, the energy field expands out to 65 miles. That acoustic recording came from the unique instrument known as a molecular scanner, which is the invention and property of an extraordinary and brilliant scientist I am acquainted with.

The acoustic addition is the molecular frequency of water. That is a mathematical algorithm consisting of frequencies ranging from zero to 32,000 cycles per second, and each of these frequencies occurs in a different sequence. The sequence can repeat, but not in precisely the same order. And this is what's called an algorithm. Since water is necessary for life, it appears that this is the mathematical formula for life and living things.

In the research I was doing with my acquaintance, he agreed to use his molecular emission scanner and see if he could pick up any kind of signal coming from the ring at a distance of ten miles. He was in his lab on top of a mountain. I stood in my backyard and holding my 3½ Cubit Ring, I very slowly scanned just over the top of the mountain, just above the skyline. The researcher could pick up a change in the frequency pattern. He was able to take a "before" and "after" reading. There happened to be a very small cloud in the sky above his lab, so I decided to aim the ring at the cloud. He took a "before" reading of the cloud. Then I put the beam on it and he said, "Oh, my gosh. It really is changing!" His instrument readings were dropping rapidly and he had never seen a reading so low. He converted his readings into an audio signal and it sounded like a fly buzzing, which is the sound of a water molecule in microwave frequency converted to audio. It suddenly smelled like ozone in his shop, which he had never experienced before. We made an audio tape and started playing it on a boom box and the air began to smell like ozone, very sweet, like a mountain meadow in the spring.

FIRST OBSERVATIONS OF THE AGRICULTURAL HARMONIZER

Our first experiment was near a little town just north of Denver. One of our more sensitive friends had just moved to a small farm and there were prairie dogs on the hillsides and real dry conditions. The neighbor who was leasing their cornfields was experiencing a lot of damage from earthworms. The soil was hard. She was an avid gardener and she said, "There are no earthworms here. I can't grow a garden when there are no earthworms. And, there are no butterflies!" So we placed a very, very crude early model of an Agricultural Harmonizer at her home. Well, being very sensitive she said, "This is too much energy. I can't sleep. I've got more energy than I've ever had, and I don't need to sleep, but I feel like I have to once in a while. It's a habit." We said, "Well okay, let's move it away from the house." So we went about a half mile up the lane there on the farm and just placed it up in the crotch of a pretty good-sized cottonwood tree. We checked back with her every few months. We went back up to visit the following spring, actually, probably in June or July. There was green everywhere. The creek bottom that had been totally barren - just nothing but rocks - was full of green, and there was vibrancy to the corn, and absolutely no insects in the corn. Absolutely none at all. She reported she had seen more ladybugs and more butterflies for pollination than there had been the year before. Her ground was more friable, more workable. It was filled with earthworms again. And by the way, the prairie dogs had moved out. They were gone. So these were just our first observations.

HARMONIZER IMPROVES AGRICULTURE CONDITIONS CREATED BY DROUGHT

Water treated with a ring starts to emit photons, and the water brings light into the soil and increases its quality. Five years ago we applied Agricultural Harmonizers and Light-Life Rings, along with an Australian device, to generate water in Northern Mexico to break a drought period that had already existed for 13 years. During that drought, they were only able to grow buffalo grass seed. Within three years, they re-established their livestock, grew pasture grass, and produced a five times greater crop yield. The rivers began to overflow and to deposit soil. This new weather pattern has been consistent now for four years of observation. In agriculture, we saw an increase in the biomass of the soil, an increase of beneficial insects, and a decrease of non-beneficial insects. This is due to the increase of light generated by the Harmonizer.

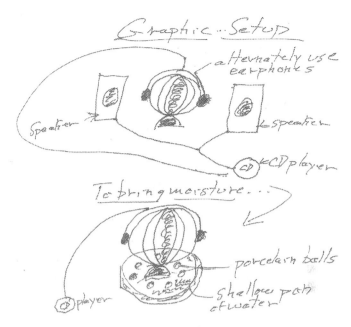

Slim recommended using this configuration to encourage rain.

INSECT CONTROL USING TENSOR FIELDS

Report on Insect Control Using Sound Powered Tensor Field, Modulated by Natural Frequency Algorithm of Water Molecule.

Experimental Proposal: To determine whether small scale observations of reduced insect pest activity and increased plant vigor resulting from application of tensor field modulation can be applied successfully to larger farm operations.

Event Sequence: In late June of 1995, McCurry received the device called the "Agricultural Harmonizer," a tensor field device with an audio tape recording of modified water frequencies. Application began on July 3, 1995. McCurry applied the field modulation unit for one to two hours, morning and evening. He noted that the numbers of corn borer millers attracted to the outside lighting on the house in the evening declined rapidly from approximately 100 - 150 millers on the window screens to "maybe" three to six. This happened in about 48 hours.

During a short absence, the unit was not operated. On his return, McCurry noted that the miller population density had returned to 100-150 insects visible on the screens.

Upon re-instituting the tensor field program being operated one to two hours, morning and evening, the miller population again declined to the five to six per screen area.

Another short trip away from the farm later in the season and subsequent non-operation and restart of operation had the same effects noted above.

Just prior to harvest, McCurry made a field survey inspection, finding only one borer per stalk. Neighbors at some distance reported 8 - 12 borers per stalk.

Results: McCurry was able to harvest at the normal ripening and field drying conditions, whereas other operations in the area were obliged to harvest early and bear the expense of spraying during the growing season and costs of drying the wetter corn in their fields.

Late Season Observations: In McCurry's area, there was a first ever observed out of season hatch of the current year's offspring of corn borers. This occurred just as the frost season was beginning. McCurry noticed also, as an aside, that ladybugs appeared in the area in great numbers, literally covering the side of his house. This was the side of the house that had the Harmonizer device operating. Ladybugs had been absent or scarce during the preceding 30 years.

Conclusions: Use of the Agricultural Harmonizer device with the audio frequencies of water for short periods during the day in the growing season can dramatically reduce certain insect pest populations. As an additional factor, beneficial insects appear to reproduce better and/or are attracted to the area. Cost savings are significant.

Prior observations related to pest and insect populations of different species:

1. Water treated with tensor field devices eliminated aphids on roses in two days when sprayed lightly on the hedge of the plants.

2. Same water liberally applied to soil in a small area in two applications produced a five foot difference in a few stems of

the bluebell ornamental species. This is compared to "normal" growth in untreated watered areas. Deeper colors in specially treated stems were noted in both leaf color and bloom color. This was for the 1995 season.

3. *Application of water frequency modulated tensor field broadcast during the '95 season resulted in intensified colors and plant vigor in local ornamental and wild flowers. Noted out of season hatch of houseflies in '94 season and significant reduction of fly population in '95 season. Leaf miners and unidentified species attacking local Siberian Elms causing sap to drip on cars in street was practically absent in the '95 season, in contrast to the previous five years without broadcast.*

4. *Tensor field modulation by audio in molecular water frequency range appears to very significantly reduce pest insect damage across a range of pest insect species and plant host species. The plant species' increase in vitality may account for the effect. Exact mechanism is not well defined; however, net results are positive.*

Comments: Application costs are low, costs savings significant. We are at the earliest stages of a new branch of science, developing a taxonomy of observed effects until appropriate terms describing the observed effects can be combed from the literature so as to avoid a meta-language incomprehensible to scientist or layman.

Iowa Farm Experiment with the Agricultural Harmonizer

The next application, experimentally, was under reasonably controlled conditions. We put a unit and an audiotape on a big corn farm operation up in northern Iowa with about 400 acres. During the week they installed it, the agriculture department at the local college issued a four-county warning about an outbreak of the corn borer. This is an insect that bores in right where the ear attaches to the stalk. The result of that is by the time harvest comes, the ear has fallen down or even fallen to the ground, and a farmer can lose two-thirds or more of the crop.

Well, the farmer had an outside light on the porch, and in the evenings, he noticed five or six hundred of these little millers, little moths on the screen of a small back door. The night after he started the audio program with the Agricultural Harmonizer, there were just five or six. They had simply disappeared. And this was an unheard of phenomenon.

He didn't have to use poisons. He didn't have to use any special harvesting technique or harvest early and dry his corn at great expense. He was able to harvest at the normal time. The crop was mature. It was dry. The following year, they went from 120 bushels to 150, and the third year he got 180 bushels. No change in his farming practices, except one: the Agricultural Harmonizer. He kept it operating 24/7 during growing season.

If plants are healthy, they're not attacked by insects. And air pollution contributes greatly to the ill health of plants by altering the solar spectrum. It lowers the natural solar spectrum and its frequency. So let's say a red would be a muddy red. A yellow would be a muddy yellow. It would be a lower frequency. The genetics of all living things have been produced under pristine skies up until the industrial revolution and the overuse of these fuels, especially with the hydrocarbon fuels. If you try to create a spectrum, a rainbow with oil droplets, your eye will instantly detect that it's not the same color as a natural water droplet-produced rainbow. And it's this filtering action of hydrocarbon vapors in the atmosphere that's lowering the vitality not only of plants, but of every living thing on the planet. So, as one farm by another, one individual by another, owns and operates one of these Agricultural Harmonizer units, we're getting rid of a little bit more air pollution. This occurs as the wind blows through that field and alters the air mass downwind of it.

We introduced one of our very early, very primitive Agricultural Harmonizers into a detox center where a chiropractor friend was treating some of the inmates. He just walked in, set the Harmonizer on the director's desk and said, "I'll be back in a little while." When he walked in, it was bedlam, men and women screaming and hollering, struggling with their detox symptoms. He said in two minutes flat, it was quiet in that building. Two minutes flat.

Sacred Cubit and Lost Cubit Personal Harmonizers

The Personal Harmonizer follows the same principles as the Environmental and Agricultural Harmonizer, but would you wear one around your neck?

No! Makes an awful big bump on your chest. Makes it hard to give somebody a hug. So my foster brother Larry was able to miniaturize the Harmonizer, as he's a master jeweler. We had a huge demand for a necklace piece from many of our better psychics and sensitives. So we miniaturized it.

I never wanted to make jewelry. That was the furthest thing from my mind. I'm too practical. But the Personal Harmonizer turned out to be quite beneficial. And what we've done is simply miniaturize it using the harmonic relationships of length, the Personal Harmonizer being a 1/8 Sacred Cubit length. The field range of the Personal Harmonizer is five to seven feet, so if you're wearing that midway on the body, it's five feet or seven feet up, outward, and downward as well.

The Personal Harmonizer is a unique combination of the Light-Life Ring and the Acu-Vac Coil in motion. The Sacred Cubit Personal Harmonizer is ¾" x ¾" in size and affects an area approximately five to seven feet around and through the body. The Lost Cubit Personal Harmonizer is the size of a quarter and affects an area approximately eight to ten feet around and through the body. Its energy field fine structure seems to exclude or significantly reduce the influences of electromagnetic and psychic energy forms. (I am very tempted to say here that it reduces the effects of electromagnetic mind control methods and the cellular damage from the high frequency microwaves of ever more prevalent cell phone antenna radiations. My personal observations tell me this is the case, but I have no validated laboratory tests on this.)

Our own personal bio-field is being strengthened and enhanced by the Personal Harmonizer's light force energies. As the Harmonizer's energy travels through us following the meridian channels, it will work its way gently through the body from head to toe - down and up - down and up. A polarity flow of body rhythms.

One of the more interesting groups that is consciously and deliberately employing the Personal Harmonizers are law enforcement groups and paramedics because they often run into very difficult situations. And I've had a number of field reports come back from police officers in California. None of them have sustained any personal physical injury since they've been wearing these. The reason for this is whomever they're confronting seems to come into agreement with them very quickly.

It takes the edge off the anger, yet allows things to be more reasonably solved and, oftentimes, without having to make an arrest. This is a very profound thing. For the paramedics who arrive on accident scenes, they seem to operate more efficiently. They're more focused, and the injured parties seem to have less resistance to being moved or treated. There's less pain and less trauma as soon as they arrive on the scene. There are whole teams that are now using Personal Harmonizers. So this is quite an event!

FIELD REPORTS FROM RESEARCH ASSOCIATES

Sacred Cubit Personal Harmonizer and Spiritual Liberation

"I received the gold plated Sacred Cubit Personal Harmonizer as a gift and, since I don't wear jewelry, set it up next to my computer (which I spend a lot of time in front of) with the Environmental Clearing CD playing continuously through a pair of ear bud style headphones. I pretty much forgot about it at that point.

"Approximately six weeks after I had received the Harmonizer, I came home from work and sat down at my computer (my normal daily routine) and had the most sudden and overwhelming epiphany: I was happy! Nothing external had changed in my life except for the presence of that Harmonizer, yet I felt a level of contentment and peace that I had not known since being a child. Somehow, I had let go of all of my pent-up emotional baggage without ever even realizing it.

"I've heard of therapy sessions with psychologists where past issues are addressed and confronted only meet with low to moderate success rates. That was not the way of it for me. Nothing was directly addressed, even internally. I felt emotionally and spiritually liberated, and the entire process happened at an unconscious level.

"From that point until now, I feel like a completely new and improved version of my old self. I am less selfish now, actually appreciating the opportunity to help and serve others. I am also much more tolerant of people who have differing opinions from my own and much less easily frustrated in general. Thank you Slim and Katharina!" *R.N., CO*

SACRED CUBIT PERSONAL HARMONIZER WITH MINI STERLING SILVER FEEDBACK LOOP

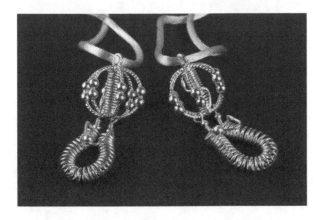

The Feedback Loop works very quickly. According to a psychic reading, "You will feel empowered when using a Feedback Loop on a Personal Harmonizer. This tool helps you tap into your mastery as an individual and manifests your self-esteem. You feel in command of your life and very grounded. This grounding centers your soul in your highest level of consciousness. Pointing the Feedback Loop away from you brings you into neutrality. Your mind goes blank. This is wonderful for a therapist, allowing him/her to remain neutral when a patient is facing them and becomes empowered. When the therapist needs to speak, he/she can turn the Feedback Loop around and will be able to effectively communicate with their patient."

FIELD REPORTS FROM RESEARCH ASSOCIATES

PERSONAL HARMONIZER WITH THE FEEDBACK LOOP ATTACHED

"I'm testing the Personal Harmonizer with the Feedback Loop attached. A customer took it into her hands to admire before I could pull back. I explained that I was testing the device and it was not advisable for others to touch it during this time. She certainly understood. Then she told me she had a migraine, and I wondered what effect that would have on me since she had just touched the device. Nothing of a negative nature happened. This tells me that the device is self-cleaning. I'm enjoying it very much!" *S.D., NH*

The Storm Chaser

The Storm Chaser came about as a result of my concern for the increasing levels of pollution, which exacerbate the natural tendency of tornadoes and hurricanes to wreak havoc. Hurricanes start off the coast of Africa as a result of the massive density of positively charged dust particles which blow off the west coast (the skeleton coast) during periodic sand storms in the summer months. These positively charged ions have a counterclockwise spin, or a negative spin. Anything with a positive charge and a negative spin is destructive to life. These charged ions tend to drag the atmosphere into a massive counterclockwise rotation which, depending on the density of charge and duration of the sandstorm, may develop into a tropical storm and then a hurricane.

As the cyclonic rotation persists, it draws in (+) charges from different levels of the atmosphere consisting of any or all of the listed air pollutants: CO_2, SO_2, NOX, hydrocarbons (all toxic materials have a (+) charge). As we have all seen on the weather channel, these storms pull in clouds and atmospheric components from hundreds of thousands of cubic miles of atmosphere. As the density of the toxins increases and (+) charges accumulate near the center, the force behind the storm rotation increases.

Based on my personal observation of atmospheric pollution in the Caribbean during a couple of flights over the area, it is far and away more polluted than any comparable area I have seen in the past 10 years, with the exception of Belgium on my first flight over that country in '97. So we can see that these storms initiated off the coast of Africa rapidly increase in strength in the Caribbean and Gulf as they pull in polluted air from the populated mainland.

These huge storms are now appearing in the Southern Hemisphere; witness the recent one in Australia called Larry, and the first ever storm off Brazil last year. This is attributed to the increasing pollution and resultant drought conditions in that hemisphere. The impact of treaties related to globalization speaks to the issues of industrialization and the increasing use of petroleum fuels in the less developed world, as well.

Having a clear grasp of what lies behind the upsurge of violent weather that is wreaking so much havoc all over the globe, I decided to develop a Harmonizer that can cover large volumes of atmosphere. While the effects of my Environmental and Agricultural Harmonizers have been well demonstrated and proven over and over again, their field radius is not big enough to handle storms of this magnitude. In order to cover the amount of atmosphere that feeds these 'Super Hurricanes' I had to invent a bigger unit. This is what led to the creation of the Storm Chaser in 2004.

To give you an idea of what the Storm Chasers are capable of, it might help you to know that right after the Katrina disaster I sent the first units to Florida where they were installed in Pensacola, Sarasota, and Vero Beach. The next unit was sent to a site near Galveston, Texas, about 200 miles inland.

Predicted to be heading toward the middle of the Florida coast, Hurricane Wilma got diverted by the Storm Chaser manned by Anthony Cowan in Sarasota. That storm hit the Keys briefly. It then scooted out to sea and took a sudden Northeastern path. Deprived of its negative ionic charge over the cooler Atlantic, Wilma dissipated rapidly, due to the high numbers of different sized Harmonizers maintained by people in our network up and down the Eastern seaboard.

Hurricane Rita was predicted to hit Galveston and inexplicably shifted to a Northeastern course, heading toward Houston instead. When it got to Houston, the eye of that storm ran into the 65-mile wall of energy produced by the dozen active Agricultural Harmonizers manned by the people in Sandee Mac's network. Rita lost her steam and collapsed suddenly a few miles out to sea.

More recently, toward the end of March 2006, a Storm Chaser maintained by my good friend Adam Trombly out in Hawaii diverted hurricanes that were all set to slam that area. They got 127 inches of rain in one week, but there was none of the predicted devastation anywhere on the 850-mile chain of islands. A great deal of damage was prevented in that instance.

These are not the first observations of the Harmonizer's effect on hurricanes. Six small units in and near Moorhead City, North Carolina stopped Hurricane Bonnie (August 1998) in her tracks. The wind velocity dropped 10 mph in the first hour the Harmonizers were activated. A great deal of damage was prevented in that instance.

There are about 60 of the Washtubs and Storm Chasers in active service in the Northern Hemisphere serving several functions. First, is to reduce air pollution levels and severe storm mitigation, secondly, to improve plant growth, and finally, to reduce soil and water toxins and improve marine environments with those reasonably near coastlines.

IMPORTANT ISSUES OF OUR TIMES

STORM CHASER

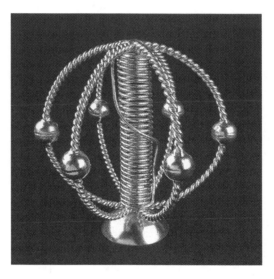

Air pollution is the biggest item on the planet right now. Since 2001, I have sold a few Storm Chasers and Washtubs, but I have given away tools to the value of $750,000 in order to have people work with them. If you have healthy trees, you don't have insects. And it is easy to have healthy trees, even in a drought. These units literally raise the water level that is in the ground. Another major problem comes with cell phone radiation. It is the microwaves and the cell phone towers that are killing the water through microwave radiation. What happens with the Harmonizer is that any frequency is instantly sent back to the source. That helps to suppress the effect of microwave radiation.

The Storm Chaser is a One Sacred Cubit Harmonizer. Slim first began sending the Storm Chaser to friends and colleagues in areas of need. The results were amazing. Slim's wife Katharina and the Light-Life Technology team are continuing his research.

It is a little bit smaller than a soccer ball and has a field diameter of approximately 400 – 800 miles when activated with the Environmental Clearing CD. [These were Slim's best estimates at the time. Ranges may vary because of increased electromagnetic fields and environmental pollution.]

FIELD REPORTS FROM RESEARCH ASSOCIATES

THE STORM CHASER AND CHEMTRAILS

"It seems that we don't get chemtrails directly over our home with the Storm Chaser Harmonizer running 24/7. We can see them off in the distance and sometimes when away from home. I am amazed at the number of chemtrails over certain areas." *R.B., MN*

OBSERVATIONS USING THE STORM CHASER

"While using the Storm Chaser with the CD running, I have observed the following occurrences: 1) Improved air quality, 2) The fires in Northern California would go out and then restart, but the fires within the 65-mile radius did not restart and seemed to go out faster, 3) An elderly asthmatic person in my home had no attacks and did not suffer from the toxic residue released into the air, 4) I ran the CD continuously during our driveway project at our home. I stated my intentions that all things go smoothly. For three days, we had perfect weather for pouring concrete. There was easy parking for all the equipment, when normally there are parking challenges. All aspects of this project were perfect. Also, my next-door neighbor has begun cleaning up the mess from his remodeling and generally getting his home in order. 5) I also sleep deeper and more peacefully with the Storm Chaser activated." *C.M., CA*

LOST CUBIT ENVIRONMENTAL HARMONIZER

The field of the Lost Cubit Harmonizer is estimated at about 100 feet in radius and about 25 miles when activated with sound. From the early reports on this new device and its energy field, it appears to dramatically reduce or eliminate either electromagnetic or psychic intrusion into one's personal environment. Interpersonal communication is improved and a general state of calm, clarity, and happiness is noted. Even plants respond very well to this energy field. The fine structure of its holographic field appears to be in accord with the primal, natural field of the planet and provides a constructive wave pattern.

FIELD REPORTS FROM RESEARCH ASSOCIATES

CRYSTAL CLEAN BEACHES

"Every winter I stay at a small beach hotel on the coast of Peru in San Bartolo, about 45 km (about 29 miles) south of Lima. San Bartolo is a long-time favorite of surfers, as the waves are consistent and the water is clean. Generally at least a couple of times a month the ocean gets "sick" as we say and turns slightly brown for a couple of days, then returns to its normal, beautiful green-blue brilliance. Perhaps it is because of the heat; I'm not sure.

"This year, however, I brought a gold-plated Environmental Lost Cubit Harmonizer and placed it in my apartment. The Lost Cubit Harmonizer is generally used to restore soil and clean water. I have only run the CD twice, but keep the harmonizer on the CD.

"Since I brought the Harmonizer here two months ago, the ocean water at this beach has remained green-blue. No brown ~ even with the heat as usual this time of year. I have seen the ocean turn brown at other beaches along the coast, but not here.

"I'm so happy to look out every day and see the waves crashing blue and green ... crystal clean!!!!!" *H.I, Peru*

LOST CUBIT AGRICULTURAL HARMONIZER

The Lost Cubit Agricultural Harmonizer seems to go out farther in its ability to radiate energy than the other Harmonizers. As it goes out into humanity, it may bring everything into harmony – thoughts, feelings, beliefs – in physical, mental, emotional, and spiritual realms. This particular Harmonizer goes into the ground, the water, and the soil, bringing in a balance of vibrations as well as changing the molecular value of the soil. (NOTE: we suggest that you test the alkaline levels in your soil BEFORE you run the unit and then again in about three weeks.) In its radius of effect, it is not only bringing humanity back into balance, but is also balancing the air, the temperature of the air, and even the cycles of the seasons within an area. Having a great number of Lost Cubit Harmonizers spread out in an area will begin to draw in creativity, productivity, and enthusiasm. These Harmonizers are also excellent for nursery and houseplants in the sense that they too will be brought back into harmony. A Lost Cubit Agricultural Harmonizer will also affect water, particularly when it is placed near a main water valve. This Harmonizer can charge the water with a higher vibration.

Slim believed that the Lost Cubit Agricultural Harmonizer is one of the things humanity needs most at this time. In its simple design, it carries an enormous power.

FIELD REPORTS FROM RESEARCH ASSOCIATES

AGRICULTURAL HARMONIZER IN JAPAN DIVERTS TYPHOON

"In 2003, a big typhoon landed in Japan. At night there was thunder and heavy rain. I started the Sacred Cubit Agricultural Harmonizer, and 10 minutes later the rain and thunder stopped. All over Japan, serious disaster happened. However, where I lived, the storm did not have any further effects." *K.S., Japan*

AGRICULTURAL HARMONIZER AND CLEAR SKIES

"We live in the Central Valley of California, two hours from San Francisco, Sacramento, Yosemite, and Fresno, which means there are a lot of particulates in the air due to all the farming and population. The color of the sky is usually a uniform blue-brown-gray, which obstructs the view of the mountains that surround us. Within a week of using the Harmonizer with the CD, we noticed we could see the mountains closest to us, and there were white clouds and blue sky! Within a few more days, we could see many other mountains that were much further away. The color of the trees and plants took on a whole different appearance. They are now sharp and bright." *J.F., CA*

HARMONIZING THE ENVIRONMENT

"I called Slim Spurling to ask for help in May 2006. The Seacoast area was experiencing severe flooding from several days of continuous rain. Slim suggested putting an Agricultural Harmonizer on top of a Storm Chaser with 12 double-terminated crystals* evenly spread around the unit. Area forecast predicted rain for another five days, and the land already had reached maximum capacity to hold more water. After turning on the CD, the rain stopped within one hour and the storm ended." *S.D., NH*

*See Appendix for a photograph of this configuration. You may copy it for your personal use.

THE DOUBLE HARMONIZERS

THE COSMIC WASHTUB, THE MATRIX 22 AND 44 HARMONIZERS, AND THE PERSONAL UNITY HARMONIZER

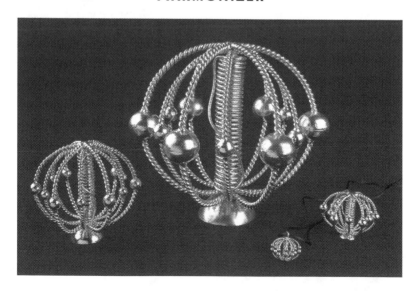

"The effect of the double Harmonizer is considerably greater than that of two single Harmonizers ~ one Sacred and one Lost Cubit ~ next to one another."

Dr. Lenny Lee Kloepper

BACKGROUND OF THE DOUBLE HARMONIZERS

Slim's intention was to clean the environment of all kinds of pollution. In the early years of the Light-Life™ Tools, Slim refrained from making 1 Sacred Cubit Harmonizers, as their energy would have been too powerful. However, after more than 10 years, communities with Harmonizers had grown steadily and, with the effect of consciousness-raising they contributed to, it was really time to come out with a more powerful version. Thus, the Cosmic Washtub was born.

Several years later, Katharina Spurling-Kaffl had a notion to create a pendant-sized Cosmic Washtub, which she named the Unity Harmonizer. One of her psychic friends told her that the name did not reflect what the Unity Harmonizer actually did. She suggested calling it a protector, as she could see the strong field that was created by this personal size Harmonizer.

The Matrix 22 Harmonizer came about when Katharina was approached to help clean the environment in a highly polluted country. It was obvious that the Washtub, although perfect for the job, was too big to get into that country. She asked her craftsmen in the shop to create an Agricultural size version of the Washtub. When tested in the field, this new Harmonizer was found to be extremely effective for that purpose. While the program in this particular country did not come to fruition, several of the Matrix 22 Harmonizers were used in a project to clean the Gulf of Mexico after the 2010 oil spill. In March 2011, several Matrix 22 Harmonizers were sent to Japan to help with radiation damage.

The Matrix 44 Harmonizer was created as demand for an even smaller version arose. The Matrix 44 contains a Sacred Cubit Environmental Harmonizer inside and a Lost Cubit Environmental Harmonizer outside. Therefore, it relates to the earth's natural harmonics in a special way. Slim believed as research progressed, this discovery would yield the secret keys to extraordinary health and extreme longevity.

All four double Harmonizers are made of twisted copper wire starting with three Sacred Cubit Rings, surrounded by three Lost Cubit Rings, and with an Acu-Vac Coil in the middle. The Washtub is made in the 1 cubit size; the Matrix 22 the ½ cubit size; the Matrix 44 the ¼ cubit size; and the Unity Harmonizer 1/8 of one cubit. The Unity Harmonizer's purpose is to protect your energy field, helping you to stay calm and centered in the midst of chaos. The larger versions' primary purpose is to energetically, as well as physically, clean the environment, water, soil, and air from all kinds of pollution.

COMBINING THE CUBITS

The Sacred Cubit as mentioned earlier, is a measurement found carved in stone as the sum of the four sides of "The Boss" above the entrance to the King's Chamber in the Great Pyramid of Giza. It has a natural resonant frequency of 144 MHz, which is a harmonic of light speed in free space. The Sacred Cubit relates to the radius and mass of the hydrogen atom and the earth. The Harmonizer's energetic pattern is like outward flowing ocean waves.

The Lost Cubit copper wire construction shows exactly 33 MHz per second increase in frequency at 177 MHz. Katharina has received field reports in the areas of natural health practice and water improvement from research associates who strongly suggest that the subtle energy bodies of living organisms can be enhanced by these frequencies.

By combining both cubit measurements into a single Harmonizer, we can achieve many of the positive effects of the Sacred Cubit Harmonizer and the Lost Cubit Harmonizer at a significantly higher level than either can reach individually.

COSMIC WASHTUB HARMONIZER

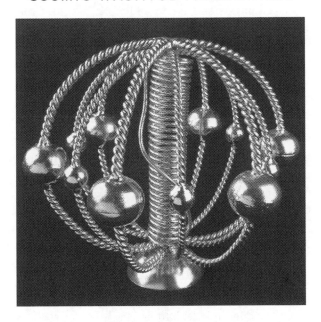

The "Cosmic Washtub" combines a One Sacred and One Lost Cubit and is the size of a soccer ball. We have about 60 units of Storm Chasers and Washtubs operating worldwide, including South America, India, Tibet, Europe, Taiwan, and the U.S. Their primary purpose is air pollution control, and thereby preventing storms from building up to hurricanes and tornadoes.

Two CDs are included with the Cosmic Washtub Harmonizer: The Environmental Clearing CD and the Bottle Brush CD. Play the CDs separately, according to the included instructions, by putting earphones around the Washtub, or by putting the Washtub in front of a boom box. Volume can be very low. Put the Washtub in the included 1½ Sacred Cubit Ring when you want to shut it down, so that its field expands only to the size of the ring.

FIELD REPORTS FROM RESEARCH ASSOCIATES

THE WASHTUB AND HURRICANE ISABEL

"I aligned a large Acu-Vac Coil with the Washtub at Hurricane Isabel as it was heading towards our shores. I monitored the intensity when it started, and the wind speed was 125 mph. For the next two days, the intensity fluctuated and then rose to 141 mph; by the time it hit shore it was 100 mph. I remembered that there was a Washtub in Florida, which wasn't hit. The hurricane squeezed into North Carolina, which is between the Washtubs in Florida and New York." *K.W., NY*

MATRIX HARMONIZERS

The Matrix Harmonizer supports life force physically, mentally, and spiritually, and may strengthen the immune system. It intensifies the six senses: sight, smell, taste, touch, sound, and intuition, and enhances thought patterns. The Matrix is believed to reduce toxic elements in polluted air, as well as assisting in clearing the earth's atmosphere. Additionally, the Matrix Harmonizer is known to balance and harmonize the aethers, harmonize magnetic and geopathic grid lines, and elevate chi force within physical structures. It seems to reduce positive ions and increase negative ions and has a neutralizing effect on radioactive material. NOTE: The degree to which the Harmonizer is able to neutralize radioactive material depends on the concentration of radioactive material and whether it is present through natural causes or waste byproduct. Regardless of the variables, the Matrix Harmonizer seems to be an effective tool in reducing radioactivity.

MATRIX 22 HARMONIZER

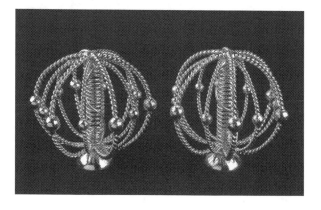

The Matrix 22 Harmonizer consists of a Sacred Cubit Agricultural Harmonizer inside a Lost Cubit Agricultural Harmonizer. It comes with

an Environmental Clearing CD, a Bottle Brush CD, and a One Sacred Cubit Ring with three beads. The Matrix 22 Harmonizer has a 'pulsing' field that seems to expand over a period of time.

We suggest putting the Matrix 22 on a sound repeater (available from IX-EL, Inc.) that is connected to a power outlet, then turn the volume down and run it 24/7 or until a situation is cleared up. Two CDs are included with the Matrix 22: The Environmental Clearing CD and the Bottle Brush CD. Play the CDs separately, according to the included instructions, by putting earphones around the Matrix 22, or by putting the Matrix 22 in front of a boom box. Volume can be very low. Put the Matrix 22 in the included ring when you want to shut it down, so that its field expands only to the size of the ring.

FIELD REPORTS FROM RESEARCH ASSOCIATES

EXPERIENCING THE MATRIX 22

"I have been running the Matrix 22 with the sound system non-stop since I received it. I moved to where I live now one year ago and am sharing a house with my landlord. Sometimes his teenage son and girlfriend are here, too. People have commented how much calmer he is, and his anger and frustration episodes have lessened considerably. People state how peaceful and calm it is all around.

"A week ago, I had a visitor (he claimed to be very sensitive) and he was very taken by the Matrix 22. He held it in his hands for almost an hour, and was very calm and relaxed afterwards. I perceived him as very intense and driven prior to holding the Matrix 22. I had to tell him that I needed to go and make dinner for my grandchildren. Otherwise, I think he would still be sitting there holding it.

"Granted, we had a very wet spring, but insects, frogs, and snakes are still out in big numbers. During our rainy season, and it was an El Nino year, damaging storms were reported about an hour away on many occasions. We had strong winds, but no damaging ones.

"I live halfway up Mt. Konrad, an old volcano. We are in the middle of a seismically very active area. I would love to get hold of some earthquake records to see if there was less activity while running the Matrix 22. There certainly were no reported earthquakes close by during that time.

"Some wonderful new people have joined our community, and very positive developments are happening here. Before, I was told, chaos was the norm. Naturally, all these things are not quantifiable and can have other sorts of reasons for occurring.

"I use my pendulum a lot and trust my dowsing quite a bit. For this testing, I used the Virtual Cone Pendulum. It is NOT used as a mental dowsing instrument, but picks up energies by the way it is contracted. It measures all the color frequencies (visible and not visible to the human eye), and you can set it for beneficial and detrimental emanations. In this system, three color frequencies are found to be very beneficial and are called the BG 3: green (not visible), gold (measured as orange), and ultra-violet. Any one is beneficial, with three being the best. My testing shows that the Matrix 22 emits all the BG 3, and none when measured on the non-beneficial setting." *C.S., CA*

Observations of the Matrix 22

"We took the Matrix 22 on our family vacation to Maine. We stayed in a cottage by the lake. In a second cottage, we were joined by a few family members. Here are some of the observations immediately felt by using the Matrix during that vacation that I would like to share:

"**Peace and Harmony:** We were playing the Bottle Brush CD approximately two to three hours a day. Animals were coming to visit, and beaver and muskrat swam directly toward us as we had coffee on the porch. We felt the silence. A loud party across the lake quieted right down. A family member chose to not have alcohol all week. Acts of kindness occurred among all of us.

"**Personal Changes:** The week before, a dear friend ended our friendship abruptly. The Matrix assisted in a speedy recovery from the shock. What I continue to feel is the wisdom of the life force. Some of the clearings that happened were very difficult, yet were needed. The Matrix is allowing me to go with the flow much more instead of fighting upstream. My need to control, to be safe, has been an issue in this lifetime. My confidence has improved.

"***Environmentally:*** My house continues to go through many home improvements. There is less procrastination. I have no problem with ants inside the house anymore. Winter was gentle here. Winds that were supposed to hit hard bypassed the area. Snow was in manageable amounts. Ice storms were not severe this year. I run the Matrix almost 24 hours a day. I rest it down at least once a week to let everything integrate.

"A computer chip company moved in north of the Capital District. It created hundreds of jobs in the area. Chemtrails seem to be broken up much more, not lingering as long. The air reports continue to consistently say "good." The ozone report yesterday said "moderate."

"***Working with Clients:*** So many things happen to people as I watch them evolve. I feel it has a link to their exposure of the Matrix. I use the tools in all my healing sessions, and the Matrix is also running. My psychic impressions have increased. My intuition feels clearer and sharper. There appears to be less merging with people's stuff and more ability to be there for people without taking on their emotional body.

"***Observations of Nature***: I particularly like running the Matrix with the sound repeater and the Bottle Brush CD. It seems to be the strongest connection for me. I feel that certain birds come around at particular times due to the organized fields. The plants outside are flourishing and abundant. They are fuller and healthier than last summer, with more blooms on almost everything. The grubs are not eating the front lawn like they have in past years.

"I am committed to consciousness moving forward, being in that process, knowing it is going places. The Matrix helps me to raise the bar on myself with discipline and commitment to a global planet. I hold intentions about the soil and the water being nourished and replenished." *V.H., NY*

REPORTS ON THE MATRIX 22

"Here are some of my findings in working with the Matrix 22:

"***Working with Clients:*** With several clients who aren't particularly dedicated to self-change, I have observed them getting more aligned with support for their bodies, for example, getting hearing aids, sleep apnea equipment, needed surgeries, etc. This group would never credit subtle energy support, but I quietly notice that where they had resisted intervention before, there is now a willingness to seek the help they need. I believe exposure to the Matrix is largely responsible.

"Clients who are devoted to self-change report abrupt terminations in professional and personal relationships of all kinds, and are sprouting into new zones of experience with more matched vibration. There appears to be disruption in all areas of life with a deferred result of more ease. Clients report, "I'm happier," and are encountering a fuller engagement in life.

"**Personally:** As for me, I feel like I know my own mind and heart much better. It used to take me long periods of sifting through the fog to come to clarity. Now I feel like clarity is more my ground of being. If I'm not clear, I recognize it and know to hold off on speaking or making decisions until clarity comes.

"My current understanding of harmonizing has more to do with respecting my own experience and the intelligence of the universe vs. an ideal of love and peace. For example, I have a difficult neighbor for whom I used to bend over backwards to keep the peace. With the Matrix in my life, I now feel outright hostility for this person and appreciate that there is no pretense of friendliness. The hostility is honest and real.

"I used to tend toward lethargy and depression. I no longer feel depressed and have energy all day long and into the night. I am happy to be alive and receptive to orders. I am less inclined to make choices based on my own preferences.

"I am more inclined to be still at times vs. being in constant motion, and naps are my friend. Self-care, in general, is a skill I'm cultivating. There is less cowardice and laziness and hiding out, and more participation and curiosity about what the design of life has in store.

"I am feeling less overwhelmed. I am more resilient and able to meet obstacles as they come along. I take pleasure in celebrating the forces of transformation working inside me. Fear doesn't stop me in my tracks like it once did. There is an increased awareness about the value of my influence, speech, input, actions, and ideas. New people and new enterprises are coming into my life, as well.

"**Nature:** Is nature moving closer? Some shift is happening where I notice the song birds are singing, one of the resident lizards is missing her tail, the red ants have moved on, the corn has doubled in height overnight, flickers come down from the trees and walk on my grass, and breezes are delicious companions. Previously empty birdhouses are now occupied.

"The previously ornamental apple tree appreciated for its blossoms these past 19 years has decided to produce apples. Plants are bountiful in general. Pigeons aren't overwhelming the property; in fact, they hardly land.

"**Environmentally:** I don't have a baseline for soil, water, and air pollution, so this is a hard area to access. Santa Fe skies are stunningly beautiful and there is no smog. I have concern for the insidious effects of radiation from Los Alamos on the soil, the Rio Grande, the air, and the health of human beings. It was suggested to me by a medical astrologer that I leave the area. With the Matrix living here, I feel confident to stay.

"Three forest fires are underway. I suspect the smoke would be worse without the Matrix running. We had an abnormally wet winter!! Hurray!

"A community garden project is underway in my neighborhood. It's been a vacant lot for decades. I am ever-grateful for the beauty and power of the Matrix in my life!" *S.H., NM*

MATRIX 44 HARMONIZER

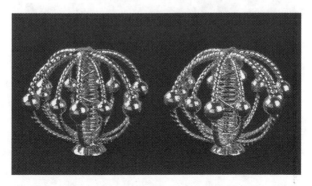

The Matrix 44 contains a Sacred Cubit Environmental Harmonizer inside and a Lost Cubit Environmental Harmonizer outside. This Harmonizer comes with a ½ Sacred Cubit Ring and an Environmental Clearing CD.

FIELD REPORTS FROM RESEARCH ASSOCIATES

MATRIX 44 RESTORES HARMONY

"I brought a Matrix 44 unit into my workplace after much turmoil and cleared the room, noticing peace and harmony were restored within 30 minutes. The owner calmed down and customers reverted to their friendly manner. Change was most noticeable. Fabulous result!

"After my experience with the May 2006 flooding incident, I placed the Matrix 44 on the Storm Chaser inside a 1 Lost Cubit Ring directly over a mapped area of the oil spill off the coast of Louisiana. I am hoping for a positive effect. Time will tell." *S.D., NH*

UNITY HARMONIZER

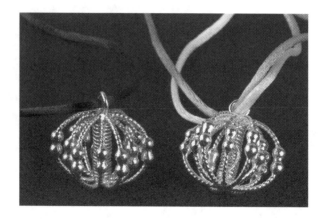

The Unity Harmonizer is the size of a quarter and is constructed with a Sacred Cubit Personal Harmonizer inside a Lost Cubit Personal Harmonizer. It holds the frequencies of the Sacred and the Lost Cubit, and so we call it "Unity." The Sacred Cubit seems to work with physical issues, while the Lost Cubit influences mental and emotional issues. It has an effective radius of about 10 – 15 feet.

This Harmonizer comes with a cord in order for it to be worn as a necklace. Also included is a ½ Sacred Cubit Light-Life Ring. It is suggested that you put your Unity Harmonizer in the ring at least once a week to clean it.

CHAPTER 10

FIELD REPORTS FROM RESEARCH ASSOCIATES

DIFFERENCES WITH THE UNITY HARMONIZER

"The first tool I ordered was a Unity Harmonizer. After about three weeks of wearing it, I found a discernible difference in my attitude towards others. I felt that I had noticeably more compassion and acceptance of the foibles of others. I realized that I was having forbearance and acceptance of those traits for which I usually had little patience. I was bemused to recognize that I had, at one time or currently, also possessed those very traits. Also, I have noticed my intuitive abilities are amped way up beyond anything I've had before." *M.M., OR*

UNITY HARMONIZER HELPS TO RAISE THE CONSCIOUSNESS OF THE PERSON WEARING IT

"It feels like you're not gonna get robbed wearing this thing. You're physically protected from people coming into your field when wearing a Unity Harmonizer. When I'm uncomfortable going into a business meeting or having to speak on stage about something controversial, I tend to put up a lot of shields. Wearing a Unity Harmonizer gives me a "Don't mess with me, I'm in my power" kind of feeling. For the energy that it has, it feels like "unity" is not actually well suited to the name of the frequency that I'm feeling, but what I'm getting is - protection. This is your protection harmonizer. That's what it feels like energetically. This would be a really good Harmonizer for everybody to have in their house, their car, and their suitcase when they travel. You may want to market it as a Protection Harmonizer. Its frequency is very clear as a protection shield. I get a high frequency, and then a sense of feeling that I need a break from it because the frequency is so high.

"The Unity Harmonizer allows an individual's consciousness to rise above, and it helps their brain waves come into calmness. It begins to slow down the brain waves, although not so slow that one cannot think. It begins to radiate a frequency or vibration that allows individuals to see things that are frightening to them in a different perspective. This personal size Harmonizer helps people remain neutral and calm and at an elevated energetic level. It allows one to hear their divine voice much louder. It seems to raise the consciousness of the person wearing it, as

155

reducing pain, and many other applications when not being used with the Harmonizer.

The coil in the center of every Harmonizer acts like a vacuum, drawing the atmosphere up and around the Harmonizer and back through the bottom. This demonstrates its toroidal field effect.

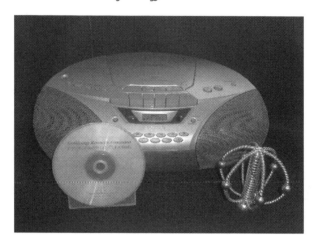

CHAPTER 11
Remove Pain without Needles or Medication ~ The Acupressure Tool

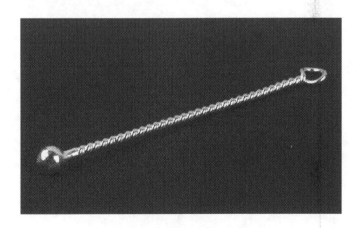

"According to my best estimate, by placing this unique antenna on the acupressure points, the proper frequencies are re-introduced to the system and amplified by the tool, thus re-establishing the proper frequencies and deleting incorrect ones."

Slim Spurling

BACKGROUND OF THE ACUPRESSURE TOOL

The Acupressure Tool is a concept brought to us by Dr. Dora Lofstrom, a naturopathic doctor in San Diego. It is a ¼ Lost Cubit in length. This length is a harmonic antenna, which is activated by the natural function of the standing gravity wave of the planet and the Schumann resonance of 7.86 hertz. The Schumann resonance is for building and maintaining the DNA and resultant physical structure of living organisms.

PURPOSE OF THE ACUPRESSURE TOOL

This unique antenna seems to delete the incorrect frequencies while amplifying the proper ones, reintroducing them to the system when placed on the acupressure points. One end can be used to stimulate an acupressure point, the other to sedate. The Acupressure Tool incorporates the benefits of the Light-Life™ Technology. We have found it eases tension, increases blood circulation, and heightens the body's vital life energy to aid healing. It is ideal for those who are uncomfortable with the use of needles in traditional acupuncture. This tool is frequently used on animals, especially horses, with great success.

DESCRIPTION OF THE ACUPRESSURE TOOL

The Acupressure Tool is 24K gold plated copper, and a quarter Lost Cubit (six inches) in length. The energy flows in both directions in the tool. It balances the acupressure points. The loop seems to concentrate life force energy when used for two to five seconds on the skin. The ball seems to create the flow and reactivation of life force energy. According to my best estimate, by placing the Acupressure Tool on the acupressure points, the proper frequencies are re-introduced to the system and amplified by the tool, thus re-establishing the proper frequencies and deleting incorrect ones.

APPLICATION OF THE ACUPRESSURE TOOL

Apart from using this tool on the acupressure points, it may also be used to remove blockages in the veins. Practitioners have used the Acupressure Tool in a weaving motion over damaged skin to repair it. I recommend using the bead for weaving the loop when removing blockages. The law of two magnets – when brought together, they either repel or bond – is similar to the way the Acupressure Tool functions. Working on the basis of opposing forces, the loop draws in, the bead pulls out.

FIELD REPORTS FROM RESEARCH ASSOCIATES

Energy Applications

"I use it personally on the third eye, on the temples, and the chakra points. Sometimes I just touch the spot, other times I let the ball lay on the area for a few minutes during a meditation. Since the Acupressure Tool is made from the Lost Cubit, it may have the tendency to heal spiritual, emotional, and mental issues, as well as the physical.

"I sometimes lay an Acupressure Tool on a Sacred Cubit Ring to infuse the Lost Cubit energy into that space. You can do this under a mattress or pillow to help mitigate discordant emotions and psychological problems. The person will awake with a greater feeling of well-being. May take some time doing this repeatedly for deep issues.

"I make the infinity symbol with it and use it throughout the aura. It seems to be very good for the chakras - opening, spinning in the 'right' direction; and spinning faster (for age reversal). Just by intent, let the tool know what you want it to do. Then use it like a magic wand circling the way the chakra spin is to go, opening up the portal with a circular motion, spinning it very fast to increase the speed. I use it with my pendulum to find out what is happening in the chakra areas, and then use the tool to 'repair' it. Then I check it with the pendulum. Has worked every time!

"Reiki masters and energy workers could use it during the attunement process to accentuate the power flow and openings. I would also suggest they wear the ½ Cubit Rings on arms or forearms. The ½ Sacred Cubit Ring size fits the arm/wrist. The ½ Lost Cubit Ring size is a bit larger, so it fits the forearm. It increases the power flow 400 times, and they may find their students realizing more powerful attunements to their benefit!" *Anonymous*

Acupressure Tool for Horses

"When I use the Acupressure Tool on horses, I begin a session off body. I will run the bladder meridian first and 'look' for any areas of blockage, heat, or sensitivity. These areas of discomfort often are identified when the Acupressure Tool moves away from the horse's body as though it is being pushed by the underlying energy, or it is pulled into a point. Typical reactions of horses are to relax immediately when the Acupressure Tool is used on their body, to move into points or areas they desire more work to be done, or to exhibit a variety of 'reactions' to feeling their energy move (becoming unblocked) including licking, chewing, passing gas, etc.

"I have used the Acupressure Tool on many horses and have found a consistency of response. It's a great tool to add to your acupressure session. Some horses prefer the Acupressure Tool to finger pressure some days, and on others, they seem to enjoy the hand-to-body work more. It's great to have both, and I take my Acupressure Tool on all horse sessions." *N.Z., CO*

Scar Repair

"I used the Acupressure Tool on a scar from a hamstring and adduction release surgery that took place four years ago. There was residual scarring and puckering. The scar noticeably flattened and smoothed out in 15 minutes. The mother of this child immediately bought an Acupressure Tool!" *A.A., IL*

CHAPTER 12
It's All In Your Head! ~
The Nose Mask, Horse/Head/Face Mask, and Eye Mask

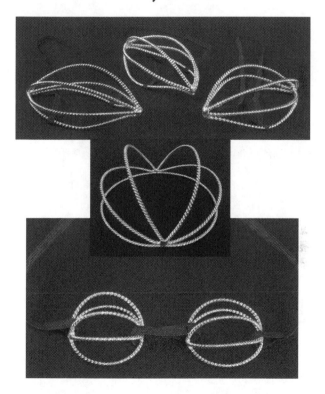

*"The Nose Mask may be the answer to many
allergic and respiratory reactions."*

Slim Spurling

*"The Eye Mask may not only help with improving your
eyesight, but also in eliminating headaches."*

Katharina Spurling-Kaffl

BACKGROUND OF THE NOSE MASK

The inspiration for the Nose Mask came as a result of a prophetic dream by a gentleman in Salt Lake City. In this apocalyptic dream, the survivors were wearing a device we now call the Nose Mask. This tool incorporates the same principles of quantum physics and sacred geometry that lie behind all of the tools.

PURPOSE OF THE NOSE MASK

The Nose Mask seems to ionize the air breathed in when placed on the face. It seems that the copper puts off negative ions, which in turn are positive for the body. Breathing through the Nose Mask can be compared to breathing in cool ocean air. It may also help the wearer breathe easier. Individuals with allergies have found great relief using it.

DESCRIPTION OF THE NOSE MASK

The high current generated in the superconducting ring incorporated into the Nose Mask causes copper ions, or monatomic copper, to sublimate from the wire. Either of these forms of copper ions is toxic to poisonous bacteria, fungus, and mold that filter down from pollutants in the air or from other sources. The copper works to kill the organisms directly, or it neutralizes the plus or minus charge by filling the "docking port" that enables the bug to attach to a cell wall of opposite charge and then interrupt the normal function of a healthy cell.

Skin carries a slight voltage generated from heart, sound, pulse, and infrared body heat. In contact with the skin, the slight voltage coming from the body and the galvanic action of sweat reacting with the metal, charges the mask in a beneficial way. When copper is exposed to water, it oxidizes, and the moisture from the skin and the breath trigger a chemical reaction as it comes into contact with the copper. The energy created may produce ionized oxygen. With every inhalation, the ionized oxygen is ripped off the copper and sublimated copper ions are inhaled with it.

The Nose Mask comes in two sizes, one for adults and one for children. It can be worn for any length of time, or for as long as it takes to experience relief.

APPLICATION OF THE NOSE MASK

Worn on the face, the Nose Mask is used to alleviate sinus problems, asthma, allergies, hay fever, or any type of respiratory ailment. Head cold symptoms often disappear soon after this device is strapped on. In areas where pollution levels are high, and on days when chemtrails are being sprayed, the Nose Mask offers both protection and relief from the effects of chemicals in the air. Come to find out, there is a fungus, a bacteria, and a mold that are resistive to antibiotics coming from chemtrails. It has been found that copper ions coming off the mask kills all three. The fungus, bacteria, and mold infect the lungs and mucous glands. Sugar is a food source that causes protein chains to grow rapidly in the mucous lining in the walls of the lungs. This is not a cure, but a remedy, and possibly a preventive measure, when chemtrails are being sprayed.

BACKGROUND OF THE HORSE/HEAD/FACE MASK

The Horse Mask came out of a necessity for an employee of IX-EL, Inc. who needed help with her horse. She asked Slim if he could make some kind of mask for her horse who was sick and having difficulty breathing. Slim created a mask for the horse, and the animal's health was restored after being treated with this new mask.

PURPOSE OF THE HORSE/HEAD/FACE MASK

The purpose is two-fold. The mask assists horses with breathing difficulties when put around their noses; for people, it is useful for those who need support in balancing their brain hemispheres, or for wearing over your face to bring some relief to congested sinuses.

DESCRIPTION OF THE HORSE/HEAD/FACE MASK

The Horse/Head/Face Mask is made out of three Lost Cubit Plain Jane copper Light-Life Rings soldered together.

APPLICATION OF THE HORSE/HEAD/FACE MASK

Given the success of using the mask on horses, the potential for an application for people had to be considered. It was determined that when the mask is worn horizontally on the head with the soldering points above the ears, the brain hemispheres are balanced. Some people reported that when wearing it vertically with a soldering point towards their third eye (space between the eyebrows), their third eye felt more open and active. This new mask was called a Head and Face Mask, since its application became so beneficial for people.

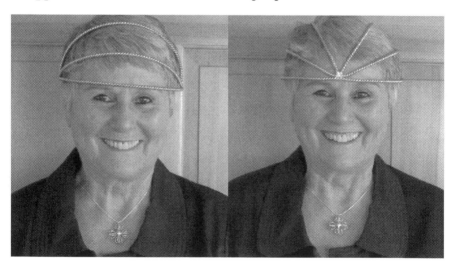

BACKGROUND OF THE EYE MASK

During a workshop Katharina Spurling-Kaffl held in Thaining, Germany, one of the participants, a 13-year old boy who had some eye problems, used the Nose Mask by placing it over his eye. Fortuitously, during this workshop, a gentleman from Belgium was present with equipment that was capable of scanning every part of the body. He took pictures of this boy's eyes before he used the Nose Mask and then afterwards. Significant improvement was noted! This gave Katharina the idea to create an Eye Mask, as she was looking for a means to improve her own eyesight, as well. What she found, and was later confirmed in reports from customers, was that eyesight did improve with use of the Eye Mask.

PURPOSE OF THE EYE MASK

The Eye Mask was designed to help improve eye sight.

DESCRIPTION OF THE EYE MASK

The Eye Mask is made out of copper wire, silver plated, with an adjustable elastic strap.

APPLICATION OF THE EYE MASK

Early reports indicate that when wearing the Eye Mask, the optic nerve and the eyes relax quickly, therefore preventing possible headache. Research associates also report amazing results with alleviating migraines within minutes after putting on the Eye Mask.

FIELD REPORTS FROM RESEARCH ASSOCIATES

HELP FOR CATS

"I have two cats. If I have a client come in that is allergic to cats and starts to show allergy symptoms, I put a Nose Mask on them and place a 3½ Cubit Ring under their head and chest (they are lying down for their treatments), and they enjoy a session without any allergic reactions." *A.A., CA*

Head Pain Relief

"Just a note to let you know how hot and humid it has been here on the New Hampshire Seacoast these past few days. I woke up with severe head pain this morning due, I assume, to a high pressure system. We are having hurricane warnings. I decided to try using the Nose Mask to ease the pain. I moved it up on the cheekbone to clear the sinus area. Within 10 minutes, all pain and discomfort was gone. In the past, I have suffered for hours, and even days, with this condition. Most Amazing! I will repeat this procedure if any head pain shows up in the future." *S.D., NH*

Help With Allergies

"The Nose Mask has helped some people with hay fever-type allergies, including my mom and sister and a friend in California, who had asthma on top of hay fever. I have used the Nose Mask when recovering from the effects of chemical spraying. Breathing through the Mask, I noticed that the cilia in the lungs was excited and moved the mucus out very rapidly without having to cough a lot. When I did cough, it was very productive, pulling mucus from the deepest parts of my lungs." *Anonymous*

A Mask for my Horse

"It has been my experience that even horses have breathing problems because of an allergic reaction to something they have eaten or an injection. This occurred when my horse had a reaction to something she ate, according to my vet's best guess. She was sweating profusely, having a very difficult time breathing, and was obviously in distress. After working with her for a long time, the vet professed there was not anything else he could do. He suggested I take her to the University Vet School for emergency surgery or let her die. Well, letting my horse die was not an option I could accept. The next day in the office, I asked Slim if he could make a nose mask for horses. He fashioned it after the human one, but larger of course. I attached the nose mask to her halter and stayed with her throughout the night. Within two or three hours, she had calmed down, was able to breathe almost normally, and was no longer sweating. By morning she was back to normal. I now keep one of these masks in my tack room because you never know when a horse is going to need help. I have not needed the mask again, but it's reassuring to know I have one for an emergency." *J.T., CO*

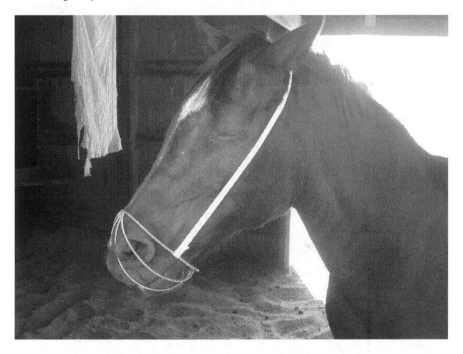

THE EYE MASK FOR HEADACHES

"Over the course of my life, I have had many headaches that come on with immediate and severe pain. Luckily, they only last a few minutes before receding again, so I have just come to accept them as a matter of course. Recently, I was conversing with a co-worker when one of those headaches struck. I stopped speaking in mid-sentence and inhaled sharply through my teeth while pressing a palm to my temple. She asked what was wrong, of course, and I explained about my headaches and how I would probably be fine in a few minutes. "Here, hold these up to your eyes," she told me, and handed me a pair of eye masks. I did so, and all traces of the pain instantly vanished. Wow! I think I just might want to keep a pair of these things close at hand from now on." *R.N., CO*

CHAPTER 13
Increase Your Vibration on a Cellular Level ~ The Seed of Life and The Lotus Pendant

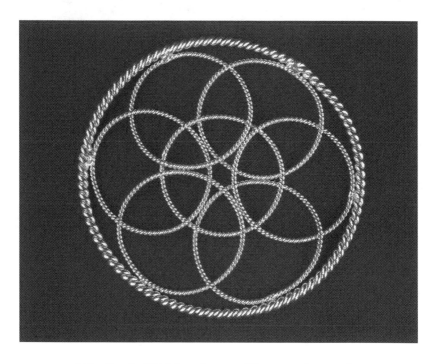

"The Seed of Life has been a life saver for my dog, Little Bear."

Tana Blackmore

BACKGROUND OF THE SEED OF LIFE

The Seed of Life was originally designed in this format for our friend Tana Blackmore's mother, who was experiencing severe health problems.

PURPOSE OF THE SEED OF LIFE

It uplifts the consciousness into higher mind states where all is released and forgiven, knowing that with this clarity you can see the good in all your life. This is very good for individuals who get caught up in mental anguish and do not remember the source of love they were created in.

DESCRIPTION OF THE SEED OF LIFE

The Seed of Life is a configuration of eight rings created in two different styles. The first is made with seven 24K gold plated ½ Sacred Cubit Rings inside a 24K gold plated 1 Lost Cubit heavy Ring. The second is made with seven 1 Sacred Cubit Plain Jane Rings inside a 2 Lost Cubit heavy copper Ring.

APPLICATION OF THE SEED OF LIFE

Hold the Seed of Life with your arms around it at the level of the heart, and connect with it. It is essential that it be at the level of the heart. The Seed of Life is used for healing by raising the vibration on a cellular level. When the vibration is higher, there is less pain.

I created the Seed of Life in order that humanity may know their own personal truth. Each of us faces struggles that do not allow us to clearly hear our truths due to negative judgments and the learned behavior of holding oneself down. As an individual encounters the energy from this configuration, there is a gentle inward reminder that humanity is not created falsely.

The energy seems to flow out of the ring, expanding to approximately three times the size. The closer the body is to the tool, the stronger the energy. Rubbing your hand quickly back and forth across the Seed of Life in a straight motion helps to balance and clear the energy before each use. Do not go in a circular motion, so as not to disrupt the matrix. Moving the Seed of Life slowly up and down when concentrating on a specific area puts the energy into motion and seems to kick it up a notch. We found that the Seed of Life works extremely well in healing sessions. We are getting a lot of positive feedback from users of this tool and continue to research its potential.

FIELD REPORTS FROM RESEARCH ASSOCIATES

MOTHER AND HER "STAR"

"I got the call from Mother shortly after she left the emergency room with a diagnosis of double pneumonia and a strong recommendation to be admitted immediately. She was calling from the ranch, an hour's drive from the hospital. She said not to worry, she was going to bed, and I didn't have to rush home. I was in Colorado on business. I called Slim to see if he had any special magic for her and, thank goodness, his place was on my way. Slim was always my hero, and this time was no different. He handed me one of the prototypes of the Seed of Life units and another strange thing he had just come up with. It looked like a wire cage shaped like an oxygen mask, with a light elastic strap tied on. He said, "Have her breathe through this, and it should make a world of difference." It did! When I arrived home, Mother was truly very ill and weak. She also had huge, red, and grossly swollen fever blisters all over her nose and mouth. She held the Seed of Life over her chest, and we placed the "mask" over her nose and mouth just like an oxygen mask. Of course she was on antibiotics and every natural medicine I could get down her, but she just wanted to sleep, and did for nearly 24 hours.

"I was in the kitchen fixing breakfast trying to be quiet, when Mother walked around the corner. It was the first time I had seen her in bright sunlight, and I was shocked! She had good color and smiled and said she felt good enough to help out with dishes at least. I could not take my eyes off of her face ... the fever blisters were small scabs and all the swelling and redness were gone! These things usually take weeks to dry up. Mother did not stay up, as we all drove her back to bed. Mother takes forever to get over these kinds of illnesses, but not this time. She got plenty of rest and we did give her lots of love, but she was up and dressed within two days. From that day forward, she literally went nowhere without her "Star."

"She went on to discover that placing the Seed of Life over any painful area helped immensely, and any injury healed in a fraction of the time. If you are wondering why Mother kept the Seed of Life tucked in her pants, well, she had digestion problems and her "Star" fixed all the bloating, pain, and discomfort she felt when she ate. We love to use this tool after big meals when we have overeaten. After a few minutes, you are comfortable and ready to go. I also "never leave home without it." *T.B., MT*

LITTLE BEAR

"Where was Little Bear? We had just finished our water and wildlife survey and were headed back up a steep ravine, high on the mountain. Little Bear was a 'coydog' (half coyote), tall and lanky, who loved to run and would cover miles in a day. We decided to take off without him, knowing he would easily catch up as we bounced slowly over the rough terrain. As we stopped at the first gate, I turned and saw the dark figure coming at a slow run to catch up. Something was very wrong, he was struggling and his head was down. Then I caught sight of the foam and heavy saliva pouring out of his mouth. I reached down to lift his chin to get a better look, and his entire neck was swollen like a massive pouch. I knew what had happened -- snake bite. My heart lurched; he had just pumped all that poison through his system trying to keep up. We were miles from the ranch house and an additional hour to the nearest vet. Bear collapsed into the lap of my friend Denise in the back seat, and Mom began to pray as I recklessly began our flight off the mountain. Bear was crying with pain and then went quiet. Still miles from home, Denise begged me to stop and say goodbye to Bear. "Tana, he is dying there is almost no pulse anymore. His heart has nearly stopped." I should be used to country living and all of the perils, accidents, and loss of life it brings, but this was still unacceptable.

"My mother suddenly looked at me and said, "The star!" She reached under her shirt and trousers where she usually had what is now known as The Seed of Life. Denise placed the 'star' over Bear's heart, checking for a pulse, while I bounced us down the mountain. Within a minute, I heard her soft voice, "I can feel his heart again." By the time we reached the ranch house, Bear wanted up and tried to jump out of the vehicle.

"We gave him Rescue Remedy and a couple of homemade tinctures of

Hawthorne (for the heart) and Hound's Tongue (an old Native remedy for snake bite). I called the vet and begged him to stay open.

"An hour plus later, we arrived at the vet's, and Bear was almost hard to contain. He jumped out of the truck and we herded him into the office. My friend, the vet, looked at me and inquired if this is the deathly ill snake bite victim. Then he asked if this was a growing abscess that I simply hadn't noticed until now. Meanwhile, Bear was running around, evading our attempts to catch him and get him on the table. We showed Doc the bite marks and he said, "Well I'll be, he should be in pretty bad shape by now. That swelling should have blocked his throat. He is lucky to be alive." Bear was still whining and crying pitifully, but wanted no part of this place. Doc said that these bites were extremely painful.

"Bear received his shots, a lot of praise, and had a miraculous recovery over the next couple of days. Of course, he slept with the star and wore a ring around his throat, too." *T.B., MT*

THE LOTUS PENDANTS

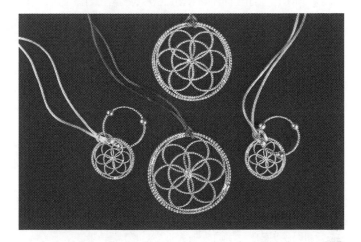

"The Lotus Pendant is beautiful, as well as being a powerful tool for raising your energy on a cellular level."

Audrey Cole

BACKGROUND OF THE LOTUS PENDANT

The idea for the Lotus Pendant came from the Seed of Life. Katharina Spurling-Kaffl and her team were looking to create a more personal use of the Seed of Life. Knowing a pendant could be worn on a daily basis, the Lotus Pendant was born! It was named the Lotus Pendant because it reminded Katharina of a lotus flower. The first creation was a ½ Sacred and a ½ Lost Cubit Lotus Pendant however, for some, it was too heavy to be worn around their neck. The craftsmen at IX-EL, Inc. then created a ¼ Sacred and ¼ Lost Cubit Lotus Pendant.

PURPOSE OF THE LOTUS PENDANT

The Lotus Pendant seems to create harmony out of chaos. It calms and quiets the internal being allowing the person to come into Oneness.

What is true for the Seed of Life is also true for the Lotus Pendant. It has been referred to as the "Soother of the Soul" and is powerful in supporting your healing and transformation on a profound level. According to reports from our advanced healers, the Lotus Pendant is one of our most potent personal healing tools.

The Sacred Cubit Lotus Pendant seems to realign polarity. It uses fractal energy to transform a person closer to the perfection and harmony of creation, both at a cellular and a spiritual level. It corrects what is out of harmony, out of configuration, out of frequency, or out of vibration, and aligns it according to what is correct for the person wearing it. Also, it can help circulate energy in a space where it may be stagnant or stuck. When placed under a container of water, the Sacred Cubit Lotus Pendant changes the molecular value of the water. Water left over acts as "mother water" when refilling.

24K Gold Plated Sacred Cubit Lotus Pendant

According to some of Slim's research associates, the 24K gold plated Sacred Cubit Lotus Pendant seems to reset and harmonize DNA. This pendant raises core vibration after about 30 days of wearing it constantly, enabling the body to respond with a stronger healing energy. This is good for people working near synthetic or electrical material. The 24K gold plated Lotus Pendant supports masculine energy.

Silver Plated Sacred Cubit Lotus Pendant

In addition to having the same properties described above, the silver plated Lotus Pendant is good for anyone who is energetically sensitive or is an empath. Wearing this pendant may also help balance their chakras so they are not taking in too much energy. Those who describe themselves as shy and retreating, or who feel uncomfortable in social situations, should benefit from wearing a silver plated Lotus Pendant. Several clairvoyants and medical intuitives have stated that it takes up to 60 days of continual use for the full effect to be realized. A person wearing the Lotus Pendant may notice that it refines their qualities and gently opens up intuition when working on the higher level chakras. Other traits attributed to the silver plated Lotus Pendant include helping the body to experience a gentle transition, amplifying creative expression, and giving the wearer a sense of empowerment. The silver plating supports feminine energy.

CHAPTER 13

24K GOLD PLATED LOST CUBIT LOTUS PENDANT AND SILVER PLATED LOST CUBIT LOTUS PENDANT

The Lost Cubit Lotus Pendant strengthens and increases the DNA. It is activating more DNA within the DNA strands, thus increasing the DNA. Stronger than the Sacred Cubit, the Lost Cubit Lotus Pendant is perfect for somebody that has already achieved the level of unconditional love and a higher spiritual body. The Lost Cubit Lotus Pendant magnifies these feelings, which not everybody can handle. This is for an individual that works hard to experience life in a loving and unconditional way. They have healed through their fears, no longer filled with aggression or anger. The Lost Cubit Lotus Pendant is taking that filigree and re-imprinting the DNA with the original blueprint, opening up communication with it.

The difference between a 24K gold plated Lost Cubit Lotus Pendant and a silver plated Lost Cubit Lotus Pendant does not seem to be as significant as the differences between the Sacred Cubit Lotus Pendants.

DESCRIPTION OF THE LOTUS PENDANT

The Lotus Pendant comes in two measurements:

- ½ Sacred and Lost Cubit
- ¼ Sacred and Lost Cubit

It is made from copper that is then plated with at least eight alternating layers of 24K gold and silver.

Larger Size: The outer ring of the pendant is either a ½ Sacred Cubit or a ½ Lost Cubit Ring. Inside the ring, forming a lotus pattern, are seven ¼ Sacred Cubit Rings.

Smaller Size: The outer ring of the pendant is either a ¼ Sacred Cubit or a ¼ Lost Cubit Ring. Inside the ring, forming a lotus pattern, are seven 1/8 Sacred Cubit Rings. This ¼ size includes a separate ¼ Sacred Cubit Ring with three fixed beads. The beads are set to amplify the power of the Lotus Pendant. It is suggested that this is helpful as a protection against psychic attack and helps to strengthen the energy field. It is also good for pain relief. The ring and the pendant can be worn together or, initially, apart until one's personal field is fully adjusted to the effects of the higher frequencies.

APPLICATION OF THE LOTUS PENDANT

Wearing the Lotus Pendant throughout the day seems to organize the cellular structure, allowing the person to maintain a state of peace.

The Lotus Pendant seems to affect each area of the body differently. Take advantage of this pendant's native intelligence by laying the pendant on each chakra for five seconds every morning before rising and every evening before going to sleep. This seems to nourish and balance each chakra.

Another brilliant use of this pendant is to place it under the mattress of a person from baby to elderly. This seems to create a state of well-being even when mental, emotional, and/or physical disabilities are involved.

If you are sharing your Lotus Pendant with someone else, whether a partner or friend, it is important to clear the pendant between users. The reason for this is that these tools pick up a person's energy. Clearing can be done by setting the pendant inside a ring for a brief period of time or by passing it through a ring as if you were dipping it into the energy column. A few passes up and down through the ring will clear it of the previous user's energy.

Another way to clear a Lotus Pendant is to brush over it with your hand. It is suggested not to use a circular motion, but rather that you use a north to south movement, followed by a west to east sweep.

For pain relief, lay the Lotus Pendant on the area where you are experiencing pain. Wear the ¼ Cubit Lotus Pendant with the attached ring to help you if you feel you are being attacked energetically by outside influences. When you are feeling ungrounded or are having difficulty staying in your own energy, wearing a Lost Lotus Pendant is helpful.

There appears to be a directionality to the Lotus Pendant. It is suggested that the pendant be hung from a chain or its ribbon in a north to south direction. This can be dowsed to determine the correct placement.

FIELD REPORTS FROM RESEARCH ASSOCIATES

The Large Rings and Lotus Pendant Testing

"I had a woman bring her Autonomous Reflex Testing machine over. We used Kandis from my office as a test subject. She has done lots of belief work, so her energy field is quite clear, although she is at the start of rising in vibration.

"We measured her vital forces, which were 82 (quite high). Then I had her hold the 24K gold plated Lotus Pendant over her heart, and her energy rose to 320. We repeated the exercise with the silver plated Lotus Pendant, and her energy went from 82 to 110, a much smaller increase. We asked questions around whether the silver would be seen breaking up the electromagnetic fields. We consistently got a "no" answer. All answers were consistent with the 24K gold plated pendant being superior, although we may have not landed on the correct questions at this time.

"We then worked with the coil with the three balls evenly spaced, but couldn't see any discernible difference in her energy field. This is most likely because we haven't hit upon the proper usage. Certainly did not have any effect on the heart area." *J.M., Canada*

A Healer's Experiences

"Hi, I'm Doctor Lenny Lee Kloepper, although I prefer Doctor Lenny. I've been using the Lotus Pendant for about one year. I've spent 40 years helping people's bodies heal. I also have 17 years' experience with homeopathy. My degree is in Chiropractic, with certification in acupuncture and nutrition. Since beginning the use of the Lotus Pendant, I've experienced an increase in overt intuitive impressions, both in quality and quantity. As my primary healing function is empathic, this has allowed a noted increase in the ability of the healing to occur since I prefer to function, as nearly as possible, with specifics verses generalities. When first placing the pendant on the heart chakra, my initial change was one of expansive response, bigger, and more open. I've noted change in the ease of intuition since that first use. The pendant has definitely affected the other chakras, as well, by allowing a great energy to flow through them. If you're interested in love's relationship, the changes forthcoming from this pendant will allow a much easier transition from now to the future. If you are a healer, it's definitely an asset no matter which level of healing you choose, since it allows a greater and more stable flow of energy. I'd highly recommend this and any and all of the other appropriate tools suited to your needs." *Doctor Lenny, CO*

Pain Free, a Face Full of Kisses, and the Lotus Pendant

"My husband had turned off our outdoor water, so on a rather hot fall day, I was watering the plants from the rain barrel. I went beyond the necessary five buckets, to close to ten, before I was satisfied that all the plants had been soaked.

"When I fell into bed that night, my right shoulder and elbow hurt, but I was too tired to do anything about them. Soon after, darting pains shot down my fingers. A phrase popped into my mind that was not inspired by a spiritual impulse. From under my pillow, I pulled out my Lotus Pendant, spread open the ring and pendant, and set them on top of my fingers. In moments, the pain was gone.

"I then set the ring and pendant shoulder height on the bed and rolled onto my side to sleep on them. I don't know for sure who or what sponsored the next event. I experienced myself walking on a beach. It was a sunny day and people were playing in the sand and water. I heard a shout, "Hey, Kirsten!" My grandmother stood before me. She took my face in her hands and kissed me several times. She stood back and asked, "Kirsten, how long has it been?" I was too surprised to answer. "A decade!" she said. We linked arms and walked along the beach.

"When I awoke, the pain was gone from my shoulder. I then wrapped my elbow with the ring and pendant on the ribbon and fell back to sleep.

"Upon waking a second time, I stretched my right arm. There was a slight sensation in my elbow still. A decade? Yes, Grandma had passed a decade ago!" *K.S., CO*

Chapter 13

A Painful Hip No More!

"I wore my 24 gold plated 1/2 Sacred Cubit Lotus Pendant around my neck on Friday, the day it arrived, as well as the next day, too. Since it's three and a half inches in diameter, it's too large to really wear it like a pendant, but it's just beautiful and I like to stare at it. I can see some of its aura, too - like a sphere of golden white light. I think, though, that the light energies also follow its curves and bends, but so far I haven't found a viewing condition/environment in which I can see the details.

"Sunday morning I went to the store. So I stuck it in my left pants pocket. It's placed right above my left hip, which has gotten more and more painful for the past couple of years. When I got back from the store, I could get out of the car without having to wait a bit for my hip to painfully realign itself for standing vertically - or whatever it does, LOL! That pleased me. For the past year or so, by the time I'd get back from the store and lugged in all the groceries and heavy cases of water, and then put away the produce, I had no more energy. So I'd grab some lunch, sit down and then keel over on the couch and take a nap of at least an hour! BUT - yesterday I didn't need a nap and didn't realize until supper time that I hadn't had a nap! Today, also, I haven't needed a nap! And I worked straight through until about 2:15 before I decided I was a little hungry and so ate some lunch.

"My hip is so much improved. I can sit for longer periods of time. When I get up, I don't have to wait for it to realign itself. The pain, which was an ache that was there much of the time even when I wasn't moving, is gone.

"I originally ordered this tool so I could hang it in a closet in the center of the house. So, am I going to hang it inside the closet? NO! I'm keeping it in my left pants pocket until my hip is healed and good and strong again. BTW, I am 80 years old and was beginning to feel my age. But now with the help of this tool, I'm feeling several years younger! Thanks so much!" *F.D., NJ*

CHAPTER 14
Let More Light In ~
The Beyond the Sky Ring

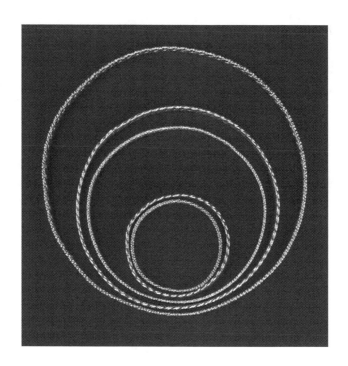

"... with these new rings, it's beyond the sky!
So, I call them the "BTS" Rings."

A Healer

BACKGROUND OF THE BEYOND THE SKY (BTS) RING

The BTS (Beyond the Sky) Ring is based on a design suggested by an alchemist out of British Columbia, Canada. Hammered copper has the surface polarity of normal copper, but which is transmitted to the interior of the metal during the flattening process. Hence, its properties include the ability to attract the nano particles (monatomic gold, silver, and platinum) from the atmosphere where they and all other metals and minerals are formed prior to aggregation into larger clusters of metal and mineral.

The monatomics have the quality of conferring health benefits to living organisms, plants, and animals by providing a micro resonance, or dance of the atoms in harmony, much akin to the music of the spheres. The micro/ nano particles are merely high density gravity spin fields, much as the planets are coarser, slower moving gravity spin fields comprised of lower undertones and longer wavelengths. When all the trace elements are in balance, they literally form a symphony of pure tones, which in fact is the creative glue that binds them together and allows for the further creation of substance to fill in the "empty space" between them. Look at the tiny amounts of metals - micro and milligrams - of trace elements in the body. All enzymes contain one or more trace element metals. Enzymes are responsible for all metabolism in the body, yet are present in tiny amounts.

Additionally, the rings generate light de novo and cause water to emit light in the full spectrum from visible to ultraviolet. Cells communicate via laser-like photon emissions in a water medium to enable transfer of DNA codes to the next generation of cells. Just place a freshly cut onion on a photographic plate for 24 hours and watch a self-portrait of the onion appear on the developed film. This is called mitogenic radiation and comes from the mitochondria of the cut cells. Fritz Popp is the German researcher who discovered this.

The purpose in having this type of ring in the hands of a select few sensitives is to conduct free-wheeling research where the preferred mode is, "What if we do this ...and see what happens?" To date, we are seeing some remarkable effects in the psychic perception area with the application of the BTS Rings to healing not only physical wounds, but also mental and emotional scars, even from long distant past lives.

PURPOSE OF THE BTS RING

The purpose of the BTS Ring is to support increased efficiency of the practitioners who have been working with the tools for an extended period of time, or for those healers who can see the energy changes occurring in the body as the tools are used. These individuals can monitor and adjust the position and length of application time of the tools during a session.

Several copies of the larger rings were sent to some of the more gifted healers in Slim's network for evaluation. One such healer emailed her observations in a few days. Very excitedly, she reported on several healing sessions she conducted with clients for whom she had been unable to resolve conditions affecting their well-being with the best of her techniques. Her comments were: "With the old rings, I thought the sky was the limit to what I was able to accomplish, but with these new rings, it's beyond the sky! So, I call them the "BTS" Rings."

DESCRIPTION OF THE BTS RING

The Beyond the Sky Ring comes in Sacred or Lost Cubit dimensions, as well as being either 24K gold or silver plated. They are constructed with twisted wire that is hammered flat. It bears mentioning that there is also a New Dimension version of each ring, as well. Please refer to Chapter 16 for more information on New Dimension Rings.

APPLICATION OF THE BTS RING

Some research suggests revitalization of the body and mind, higher consciousness levels, and increased expanded awareness. Another testimonial suggests that the BTS Rings have the highest source light that any tool can possibly bring to the planet. The BTS Rings reportedly increase the healers' affinity for work that needs to be addressed during sessions, as well as aiding the efficiency of the work. The effects of the BTS Rings appear to be more intense when held four to six inches from the body. The life force energy that is brought into the body from outside is heightened and intensified, seeming to follow the meridian channels through the body and revitalizing all parts of the body. Also, note that the BTS Rings appear to expand and increase your consciousness.

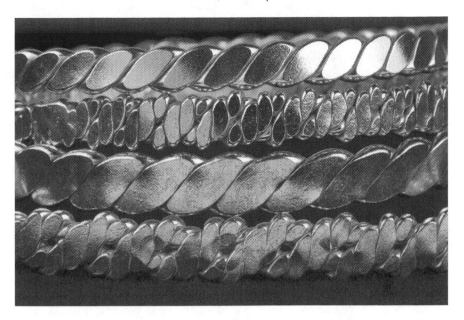

FIELD REPORTS FROM RESEARCH ASSOCIATES

A Healer's Report

"Several days ago, I did a combined session with a fellow healer on my client who has dental bridge pressure and pain in the upper cheek and face and into the head. Pressure was given as 7/10 at the start of the session. This client has a history of dental difficulties and sinus infections, as well as inner ear infections, leading to hearing loss in the right ear. I placed the large regular rings under the table and then did another overlap of the BTS Rings under the client's head. When the client got on the table and I "looked" into the field, I realized I needed to do something different with the BTS Rings as my part of the session. I changed the configuration of the rings under the table. I placed a Lost Cubit Ring directly under the head with two Sacred Cubit Rings on either side, creating an overlapping line of energy horizontally.

"I took the other Lost Cubit Ring and brought it up onto the table to work with. Now for those who may not recall, all of the rings can be used as remote viewing tools. The Lost Cubits, in particular, can be used to see beyond time and space into the past and future. I was drawn to hold the Lost Cubit BTS Ring on the side of the client's head where the pressure and pain were greatest and to look into the ring. As I stood and pointed the ring at the client's head, I looked into the cylinder and was given vivid impressions. First, I was shown a child with a huge swelling from a blow to the side of the head causing internal damage, and then I was shown a closed fist striking the head and damaging the face. I saw the energetic impressions that these events made on the energetic grid surrounding the client and how the damage to this grid had continued to spiral out of control, drawing more and more damage to it over the course of the client's lifetime. I was shown ways to disrupt this energy configuration of damage and to facilitate healing, and not just pain and palliative relief.

"I asked the client if they had experienced a severe blow to the head as a child. After a moment, they said that they had been hit on the side of the head by a piece of pipe from a playground set that had been swung by another child. The client afterward had felt sick and dizzy. I asked about being struck by a hand, and their reply was that they did not remember any such incident. I looked into the BTS Lost Cubit Ring and saw that the first strike had occurred in a past lifetime, setting up the energetic train of events for this lifetime. I had the client do some Seemorg Matrix work to clear the trauma of the blows and other connected issues, while I directed the beam of the Lost Cubit BTS Ring toward the head. Then I did some deep cranial sacral mouth work to facilitate further tissue release of the energetic signature of the trauma. Helichrysum essential oil was used to help facilitate the session. Large amounts of clearing took place. Pressure was given at 1/10 at the end of the session.

"These rings are the best, Slim! More reports as the information appears.

"I have noticed that since the BTS Rings have been with me, I have a greater affinity for what needs to be done in my sessions, and the work takes place much faster and more efficiently. My friend Carol found the effects of the BTS Rings are more intense when they are held four to six inches from the body and the energy field is directed at a specific point. She found the level of life force energy that was brought into the body from outside was heightened and intensified. When the life force was directed to an area of the body, it seemed to follow the meridian channels through the body to revitalize all parts of the body. She felt that the consciousness level of the BTS Rings was also higher and more intense. When working with the rings, her consciousness levels heightened, and her awareness expanded and increased." *D.M., PA*

Chapter 14

A Configuration of Tools

"I'd been wearing a ½ Lost Cubit BTS Ring, with an Acu-Vac Coil and Feedback Loop attached, for a few days and then added a ½ Sacred Cubit copper Ring inside the Lost Cubit BTS Ring. As soon as it was placed inside the Lost Cubit Ring, there was an immediately noticeable profound shift, a sense of rightness and comfort. I later replaced the ½ Sacred Cubit copper with a New Dimension (ND) Ring inside it, which I intuited would facilitate telepathic communication. This configuration requires a sense of humor to wear because it's a bit heavy and bulky and takes some doing to make it comfortable. Thankfully, my winter clothing masks its odd shape. After several days of unsuccessfully trying to tape these tools to each other, as well as on me, I took them off to make a pouch and sling for them to be worn over my liver. When I did, I felt a real sense of being deprived of something I didn't want to have missing from my life. At one point while making the pouch, I placed the configuration in my lap and felt my base chakra open up. After I'd made the configuration wearable, it stopped feeling uncomfortable.

"Since first writing this report, I have come to realize that the BTS Rings generate the highest Source Light that any tool can possibly bring to the planet. And, the New Dimension Rings act as a *step-down transformer* for the BTS Rings, making the Source Light more available for our 3D needs." *M.R., TN*

"Downloads" from God

"The BTS ring is aptly named ~ Beyond the Sky ~ because that is exactly what it does for me. I wear it on my head every single day because I know that I am getting "downloads" of information from God. First let me explain "how" I wear it. I like to distinguish the yes/positive side from the no/negative side because I feel that I get "downloads" quicker if I wear the BTS with the positive side down (touching my head). Would I ever wear it with the negative side down? Sure I would and I'll report back in when I do! Both sides have a positive impact. One side connects with higher spiritual realms, while the other side connects with the earth energies.

"I know some people have asked me how I know the positive from the negative. I dowsed it. As we all know, a pendulum "yes and no" answer is different for everyone. So, for me, yes/positive is a clockwise swing, and no/negative is a counterclockwise swing. So when I first received it, I dowsed it and made a permanent mark on the inside.

"Most definitely when the BTS is on my head, positive side down, and if I ask God questions about myself, my family, my friends, or my clients, I "get" answers "from above" in a stronger and quicker way.

"Why do I love going everywhere with the Beyond the Sky (BTS) on my head? The truth is I am now so used to wearing it, I forget it is there. However, I shall share some advantages that came from my "absentmindedness." (Remember, I wear my BTS everywhere: in the post office, on buses, on airplanes [after going through the check-in line], on trains, in stores, in restaurants, everywhere!)

"And now:

- People stop to ask me what is on my head and I get to share with them.

- I can be anywhere all of a sudden and need an answer RIGHT NOW and I am already "hooked up."

- Little children, especially, come up to ask me what's on my head and sharing with them is a delight because there is a part of them that already knows. I feel as if I am helping them to re-remember.

"So now I get a "tool" that is extremely useful and fun to wear. What could be better than that?

"P.S. Look how smart Slim was for inventing it and wearing it himself. He knew!" *J.L., RI*

Note from Katharina Spurling-Kaffl: Our friend who wrote this report is one of our extremely gifted medical intuitives whose vibrations are high enough to tolerate the strong energy of the BTS Ring. For people who are new to this ring, we highly recommend starting slowly by wearing it only a few minutes and then gradually increasing the time. If you start feeling dizzy, take it off.

The Magic of The Venus Mirror Finger Rings

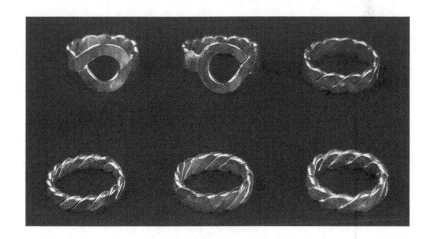

"My intent for the Venus Mirror Rings is to serve as a daily visual reminder and energetic attractor for archetypal influences that exist within us all."

Slim Spurling

BACKGROUND OF THE VENUS MIRROR FINGER RINGS

The Venus Mirror Ring is the brainchild of a friend of Slim Spurling's who suggested it, and Slim, who brought it into being. It is based on the ancient Vedic medicine concept that gold, silver, and copper have beneficial effects on physical health, emotional stability, and spiritual clarity. This is a matter for further research and investigation by the wearer.

The particular design is an outgrowth of information Slim received from a Canadian alchemist regarding the changed properties of copper when hammered. Initially, a few rings in the Sacred and Lost Cubit lengths were produced using heavy gauge twisted wire, hammered flat, and then cut to the appropriate length and bent into rings of various sizes. They were variously plated with silver or gold or left as plain copper. Slim originally made a few gold, silver, and copper Venus Mirror Rings, however as the price of gold skyrocketed, it was cost-prohibitive to continue using gold. The Venus Mirror Rings are just a tiny personalized version of the Beyond the Sky Rings. These finger rings are based on the same principles as their larger relatives.

Taking a thinly hammered section and making a wide finger ring to fit the ring finger of the right hand, Slim discovered that an unwanted emotional state dissolved in about three minutes, leaving a feeling of calm and clarity.

It was easily observed that these rings were much more potent in their effects than the same wire size rings left in the round. The clairvoyants and sensitives who saw them were ecstatic and enthusiastic at the qualities of the energy fields they observed, especially in the way they moved energy in the meridians of the body and efficiently reduced blockages and pain.

Upon direct observation, using normal vision rather than that of the clairvoyant, the inner plane of the ring is seen to be a faintly luminous sheet of energy, looking like very slightly milky glass. Under prolonged close observation, patterns emerge, especially if viewed in a dimly lit room. The clairvoyants are unanimous in their descriptions and see changing patterns and a tremendous clarity when several rings are stacked in various configurations. The Venus Mirror is an apt term for these unique combinations of metals and form.

Once the process of producing the Venus Mirror Rings was begun, the question arose as to what would be the effect of each of the rings worn on various fingers. Now it is just a matter of going to any good text on chiromancy or palm reading to determine which finger affects which area of a person's life. Further, a good acupuncture or reflexology text will yield detailed information on the meridians affecting health, emotional, mental, and spiritual states, as all meridians terminate in the fingers. After you determine which aspects you want to improve or strengthen, choose the ring which best supports your intention.

PURPOSE OF THE VENUS MIRROR FINGER RINGS

The intent behind the creation of the Venus Mirror Rings is to facilitate the development of particular traits that an individual may wish to acquire or change. Since each ring is keyed precisely to the fundamental frequencies of the wearer, they have the capacity to balance those frequencies and, depending on the metal(s) used in their construction, enhance or modify them.

We experimented and showed the Venus Mirror Rings to clairvoyants who reported that using them, they can detect unseen aspects in the aura, like root causes of illness and disease, whether physical, mental, or emotional. Their beneficial effect seems to be stronger than that of the unhammered round wire.

DESCRIPTION OF THE VARIOUS VENUS MIRROR FINGER RINGS

PRIMITIVE VENUS MIRROR FINGER RING

This ring consists of a single section of twisted, forged copper. Simple, unpretentious, and naïve, the Primitive Venus embodies the alchemical, astrological, and mythical symbol of Venus, the Venus Mirror. It also resembles the Egyptian Ankh, curved around on itself, forming a circle.

Our insightful visitor from the UK, an internationally acclaimed British healer and clairvoyant, had this to say about the Primitive Venus: "It is an excellent training ring for children when worn on the small finger. It develops sensitivity to communication with universal intelligence and helps establish and maintain contact with Spirit helpers."

Primal Venus Mirror Finger Ring

This ring consists of a single section of twisted, forged sterling silver. Simple, unpretentious, and naïve, the Primitive Venus embodies the alchemical, astrological, and mythical symbol of Venus, the Venus Mirror. It also resembles the Egyptian Ankh, curved around on itself, forming a circle.

Hidden Venus Mirror Finger Ring

Like the Primal Venus, but without the loop, the Hidden Venus establishes a "ring wall" of protection around the outer edge of the aura, shielding the wearer and insuring that those with mal-intent cannot find them. This version of the Venus Mirror Ring may be very useful for those with special gifts, knowledge, or abilities, or for those who have suffered any form of abuse.

Unseen Venus Mirror Finger Ring

This ring is like the primal Venus in sterling silver but without the loop, creating a radiant field that promotes well-being. To acknowledge the light is to have it grow and create an even larger field around you.

Evolving Venus Mirror Finger Ring

This ring is formed with one copper and one silver strand, symbolizing the development of finer attributes, compelling toward physical and emotional healing and stability. Our British clairvoyant friend's observations indicate that the Evolving Venus Ring "...can be worn on any finger. It opens and clears telepathic communication between wearers and with animals and the spiritual realms."

EVOLVED VENUS MIRROR FINGER RING

This ring is formed of one copper and two silver strands. The Evolved Venus is perfect for the individual who feels comfortable with change and wants to experience the attributes of the metals and their own archetypal energies more fully and rapidly. Again, the clairvoyant noted that the Evolved Venus Ring "...can be worn on any finger. It tempers and sharpens the aetheric communication lines within all forms of life."

APPLICATION OF THE VENUS FINGER RINGS

The acupuncture meridians follow different fingers and end right at the end of the nail, thus providing conductivity. The energy properties are related to the meridians running through the fingers. Each metal will, therefore, have a slightly different effect depending on the finger and on which aspect of your life you want to change. If you need more fluidity in your mental states and a greater range of thought patterns, first try copper, then silver on your middle finger for a week or two, and observe yourself.

The left hand stands for the past; the right hand for the present and future. Wearing a ring on the left hand would change your thinking of the past and how you perceive yourself in past situations. The thumb represents personal will; while the index finger, your business or professional approach to life, enthusiasm, and dedication. The middle finger governs the mental process that influences the career, and the ring finger is attached to the heart and emotions. Finally, the little finger governs outside relationships, the connection to groups. Copper on the little finger of both hands is worn as a protection against psychic influence. They create a ring-fence of protection against unwanted attacks.

The ancient art of palm reading instructs us that each finger is associated with a different aspect of life. According to that method of divination, the fingers conduct planetary energies. In Egyptian terminology, the God associated with each planet represents an aspect of Spirit, or 'Neter.' From the standpoint of physics, these influences are wavelengths that conduct specific frequencies into the body.

❖ ❖ ❖

My intent as a modern alchemist is for the Venus Mirror Rings to serve as both a daily visual reminder of, and energetic attractor for, archetypal influences that we have been mis-educated to dismiss as being 'outside of us' - when in fact they exist within us all. At this stage in the ascension process, it is vital that each one of us reconnect with those god-like qualities, remember who we really are, and nurture our inner divinity in a conscious way.

Beyond the hard science of medicine, chemistry, and metallurgy lies the quantum world of flux and change. Informed through thought, attention, and intention, the quantum world is full of silent sounds, of spinning waves, and frequencies of light and energy, which operate on superconducting principles – at faster than light speed. At the quantum level, time and distance are of no consequence.

The qualities of the quantum world are inherent in the Venus Mirror Rings. Each one 'mirrors' the attributes of the ancient gods and goddesses, as we do ourselves, allowing the wearer to experience the perfection emanating from their own sacred source. These rings should serve not just as a reminder of that perfection, but as catalysts for its outer manifestation. They need to be seen as custom fitted, quantum energy devices, whose practical application has to do with facilitating both the wearer's attunement to the gods and goddesses of old, and their remembrance of that which lies waiting to be reactivated within themselves.

How Do I Know Which Version of the Venus Mirror Ring is Right for Me?

The descriptions given here are my own take on the alchemical attributes of the metals based on my personal experience. My Truth may be different than yours, so call upon your inner guidance when you decide which ring is right for you. In the end, it is an individual's own sense of self and their feelings about what is needed for change, stabilization, modification, or improvement that will determine which version of the Venus Mirror Ring they choose to wear.

Copper is, in my experience, very grounding. When forged in the unique design of the Venus Mirror Ring, it is also a room temperature super-conductor which produces a coherent, life supporting, paramagnetic energy field that imparts a warm glow to the senses and clears blockages in the meridians. Which meridians? This depends upon which finger it is worn. (See a good reference book on reflexology, acupuncture, or chiromancy.) Copper holds the properties of softening and increasing communication. It cools emotions and makes ideas flow more smoothly.

Silver carries a lunar energy that is beneficial to both males and females. Silver tends to add a bit of shine and sparkle to the senses, a soft, swelling energy movement through the body, and a sense of something being purified. Energy flows with no resistance.

❖ ❖ ❖

Please bring your insights and experiences in wearing the Venus Mirror Ring to the attention of Katharina Spurling-Kaffl and to your friends and associates.

FIELD REPORTS FROM RESEARCH ASSOCIATES

WEDDING RINGS ... AND MORE

"My husband and I bought the Unseen Venus Rings as our wedding rings. I knew they would do good things for us, energetically speaking. What I didn't realize is they would help eliminate pain. I have been wearing two magnetic bracelets on my left wrist for several years now. They really helped with residual pain I have from a broken bone and surgery. While wearing the ring, I took the bracelets off, and then noticed I no longer needed them because the Venus Ring makes them unnecessary. My wrist pain is gone. My husband has problems with his left shoulder, and mentioned his pain had also decreased since wearing the ring.

"Both of us have an overall sense of well-being wearing these rings. I will definitely buy another ring in the future. All the Light-Life products are very effective and helpful. Thank you!" *D.D., KS*

CHAPTER 16
Beyond the Logical Mind ~
The New Dimension Ring

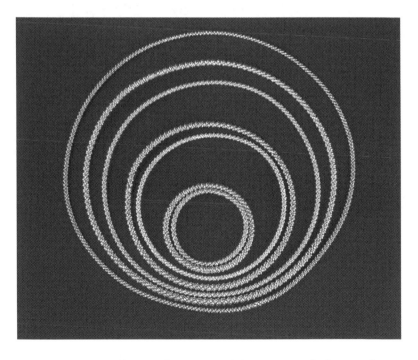

*"Let's just say the applications of this are purely for psychic
interpretation, research, and acceleration of abilities."*

Slim Spurling

BACKGROUND OF THE NEW DIMENSION RING

As I became able to spend more of my time discovering and researching over the last few years, I remembered a ring I once made. I explained the ring to an employee, and together our excitement brought us what is now called the New Dimension Ring. The ring consists of two double twists of copper based on the principle of all rings.

PURPOSE OF THE NEW DIMENSION RING

I began sending the rings out to a few friends and acquaintances for their input. The results of this research are that the rings seem to have a strong grounding of the body, while allowing the energy to flow where it is needed. The energy field of these rings seems to extend past the tensor field into the peripheral or outer edge of the rings shown vibrantly in the rings' aura. Some new reports claim the New Dimension Ring seems to create a strong energy sense of the 8th Chakra (the one immediately above the crown). The energy seems to start there and work its way down. You may feel a wave of emotions a few hours after this, as it appears to cause a cleansing and/or adjustment to happen. The New Dimension Ring appears to "plug into" the emotional and mental areas, and appears to enhance positive qualities.

DESCRIPTION OF THE NEW DIMENSION RING

The New Dimension Rings are created in Sacred Cubit and Lost Cubit measurements, as well as the hammered version like the Beyond The Sky Rings. The materials used are copper with either 24K gold or silver plating.

APPLICATION OF THE NEW DIMENSION RING

The Sacred Cubit New Dimension Ring will affect your personal life, body, and intuitive abilities. The Lost Cubit New Dimension Ring will open up to the bigger picture ~ what is happening globally, as well as what is far reaching in the universe. Intended for someone who wants to strengthen their psychic abilities, this ring allows you to see through different dimensions. I suggest wearing only one at a time, either a Sacred Cubit ND Ring on each side or a Lost Cubit ND Ring on each side.

My intention for creating this ring was to take you out of what you see as current time and space, and open up to the reality and totality of what true time and space is; to be able to go beyond the logical mind, basically, or the third dimensional properties. My intention was to have one so large that you can sit in it, put it over yourself, and as you bring it down to the ground, you are someplace else.

Give the ring to someone who is a visionary interested in activating more of their brain. If it is not large enough for them to sit in, they should hold the ring horizontally over their head. Have them flip the ring when they feel a tingling on their forehead and the back of their head. Hold the ring openhanded and horizontally moving over different chakras.

Some seers will be able to hold up the New Dimension Ring and use it for scrying where they may begin to see a vision. What I was being shown when the idea came to me to double twist the wire was that it was a sequence of simultaneous levels of reality, or what most call time and space. Instead of thinking from this brain, I would be able to use the totality of my being by undoing the density of that energy and decelerating it. I would be able to receive information from all levels of my consciousness. I was trying to create that experience, and was not sure how to formulate it and also hold the physical form. Let's just say the applications of this are purely for psychic interpretation, research, and acceleration of abilities.

You can also use the New Dimension Ring to energize water. It will strengthen the water, and you will know by the taste. If you wear the New Dimension Ring on the body, it will give you access to an incredible amount of information. It will help you with discernment and sensing out someone or something. You have to tilt it a little to achieve a 45 degree angle before you are going to be able to connect with the third eye. It works by taking internal and external thoughts and projecting them onto an ethereal screen. It increases the plasma within the human field and, therefore, the ability to see through dimensions.

CHAPTER 16

FIELD REPORTS FROM RESEARCH ASSOCIATES

A HEALER'S REPORT USING THE NEW DIMENSION RING

"My client held the New Dimension Ring in his hand and on his wrist for 30 seconds to one minute. He immediately got goose bumps up and down his back and felt a great energy flow in his meridians. The tingling and flow effect lasted for a couple of hours.

"I "see" the energy as bubbles of iridescent light. I feel like I have a pile of shimmery bubbles building on my hand when I hold the ND Ring. To me, the bubble effect means energy is "complete" and seems to carry a consciousness on where it is needed." *R.B., MN*

ARANYA'S EXPERIENCE

"When I use or carry the New Dimension Ring, I have a strong energy sense of the 8th chakra (the one immediately above the crown). The energy starts there, and then works its way down. I didn't experience any nausea, although I did experience a wave of sadness a few hours after first carrying it. I think there is a clearing and/or adjustment that happens, which is probably different.

"I have a sense that the New Dimension Ring resonates directly with Divine Will, which is why your experiences recently with manifesting worked so well. When the energies are physical and emotional, the Lost Cubit Ring steps Divine Will down to the emotional/mental levels. With the New Dimension Ring, there is no step down." *A.A., UK*

CHAPTER 17

For Advanced Healers ~
The New Dimension Acu-Vac Coil

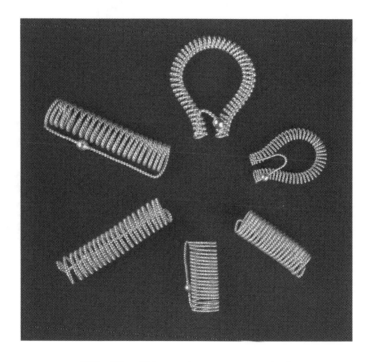

*"The New Dimension Acu-Vac Coils
are off the chart!"*

G.H.

CHAPTER 16

BACKGROUND OF THE NEW DIMENSION ACU-VAC COIL

This tool came about as a natural consequence of the New Dimension Ring. Healers were curious as to what a twisted coil could do for their healing practices. An IX-EL, Inc. craftsman made the first prototypes and they were sent out to research associates. The results were very promising! Because there are two ways of making the New Dimension Coils, IX-EL, Inc. distinguishes the differences by the making of one style with the wire on the outside, and the other with the wire on the inside. Please note the various descriptions and applications below.

PURPOSE OF THE NEW DIMENSION ACU-VAC COIL

The purpose of the New Dimension Acu-Vac Coil is to support healers in their work with clients. Sometimes the source of issues may be in another dimension or time, and this tool is of phenomenal benefit in this regard.

DESCRIPTION AND APPLICATION OF THE NEW DIMENSION ACU-VAC COIL

The New Dimension Acu-Vac Coils are created in Sacred Cubit or Lost Cubit dimension, and are 24K gold plated copper.

All New Dimension Acu-Vac Coils do the work of the standard Acu-Vac Coil, however, they have more applications, and these are described below. They seem to extend into different dimensions, as well as past life issues, and go to the source.

Sacred Cubit New Dimension Acu-Vac Coil With Wire Inside

This New Dimension Sacred Cubit Acu-Vac Coil is crafted with twisted wire. It is made with the wire and a bead soldered on the inside, similar to the standard Sacred Cubit Acu-Vac Coil.

Some research information on this coil configuration shows the approach is feminine, light, and beautiful. It seems to connect directly to the source of healing, health, light and life, and to the perfect blueprint of the person it is working on.

The Sacred Cubit New Dimension Acu-Vac Coil with the wire inside may be used to clean homes of unwelcome spirits and entities. Hold it horizontally with the bead pointing outward while scanning the area. This tool is for heavyweight issues that go beyond the dimensions. You don't want to pull the negative energies into the coil; instead, you'll enhance the positive by blasting light energy, and the negative has to go. It is almost like it is pulling you into a vortex in a higher dimension. You may feel like you're becoming invisible. You're becoming the anchor of the intention; your body becomes the intention to be cleared.

When you point the New Dimension Acu-Vac Coil toward yourself with the bead away, it helps you to remember talents and abilities you may have forgotten. It seems to activate the occipital lobe of the brain, bringing in higher knowledge of cellular memory of the things you need to know and be accountable for. With the higher activation of your brain, this New Dimension Acu-Vac Coil may bring clearer thinking and focus.

Sacred Cubit New Dimension Acu-Vac Coil With Wire Outside

This New Dimension Sacred Cubit Acu-Vac Coil is crafted with twisted wire. It is made with the wire and a bead soldered on the outside, and looks similar to the standard Lost Cubit Acu-Vac Coil.

Some research information on this coil configuration shows the approach is masculine and deep in sound vibration. It is a smooth, clear cut energy that moves rapidly, which seems to work well on the physical body.

Holding the New Dimension Acu-Vac Coil with the bead pointing towards the body at the solar plexus will help articulate what you are blocked with or what blocks your thinking. When you hold it to the heart, this tool tells you how to undo the block. When you hold the New Dimension Acu-Vac Coil with the bead away from the solar plexus, it will begin to take you out of rigid thinking and encourage the opening up of the mind.

When a person's thinking becomes too rigid, they cannot center and stay grounded. To help unblock your thinking and be more receptive to information, hold the New Dimension Acu-Vac Coil with the bead toward your solar plexus. You may get pictures or words of what is blocking you. For example, perhaps you have a fear of success, but have never been able to figure out why that is so. Holding the tool in this manner will give you an idea of why this is happening. When you then move the New Dimension Acu-Vac Coil to the heart, it may tell you what to do, perhaps in the form of a thought or an inspiration. Always work with the solar plexus and the heart chakra. The solar plexus will give you the information, and the heart will convey how to ground it into your life.

LOST CUBIT NEW DIMENSION ACU-VAC COIL WITH WIRE INSIDE

This New Dimension Lost Cubit Acu-Vac Coil is crafted with twisted wire. It is made with the wire and a bead soldered on the inside, similar to the standard Sacred Cubit Acu-Vac Coil.

Some research information on this coil configuration shows it can be used to create freedom by unblocking the mind, the spirit, and the soul and bring about wholeness. It also seems to have a very powerful female energy, and can be useful for those who feel they have a wounded soul and emotional, mental, or spiritual blocks.

The New Dimension Lost Cubit Acu-Vac Coil, when held with the wire bead towards you, seems to release trauma due to war. It has also been known to release trapped energies within the body that propagate deadly disease. In other words, it appears to be clearing from the body the limitations of life. This tool may clear your thinking, your spirit, and perhaps your DNA.

When the New Dimension Lost Cubit Acu-Vac Coil is held on your solar plexus with the bead pointed away from you, it seems to reset messages within the body contract. These messages consist of what the body is going to receive, truly allowing the body, the mind, and the spirit to become fearless. Resetting the contract to whatever your intention is seems to allow you to override astrology and numerology, and to truly live a new life in any way. If you want to set the intention strongly, move the coil up to the heart.

Lost Cubit New Dimension Acu-Vac Coil With Wire Outside

This New Dimension Lost Cubit Acu-Vac Coil is crafted with twisted wire. It is made with the wire and a bead soldered on the outside, just like the standard Lost Cubit Acu-Vac Coil.

Some research information on this coil configuration shows this is a very powerful tool, great for going far beneath the surface. It may be especially good for frightened or traumatized individuals.

Dealing in the animal realm is very similar to our human experience. For example, let's say you have a dog. Your dog feels it is their job to take pain and suffering from you. It's very difficult for an animal, a pet especially, once they've taken pain into their body, to release it. If you hold the New Dimension Lost Cubit Acu-Vac Coil with the bead pointed out under their rib cage, it will clear out anything they have accumulated from you. When the natural cycle of life has been disrupted, the New Dimension Lost Cubit Acu-Vac Coil will help to shift the imbalance and restore it.

FIELD REPORTS FROM RESEARCH ASSOCIATES

Relief from a Constant Dull Ache

"I jammed my thumb. Ouch! There was a constant dull ache with my thumb just relaxed and a considerable flare if I bumped it or tried to use it for anything. I took an Acu-Vac Coil and pushed the center wire to one side, then inserted my thumb (with the bead-end pointing away from my hand). Within just a few minutes, the ache disappeared. I left it on for about 1 ½ hours and my thumb felt like it had been healing on its own for a week. I was even able to use it (carefully) without any pain. What a difference!" *R.N., CO*

CHAPTER 18
Simple Protection from EMF ~
The Phone Ring Set

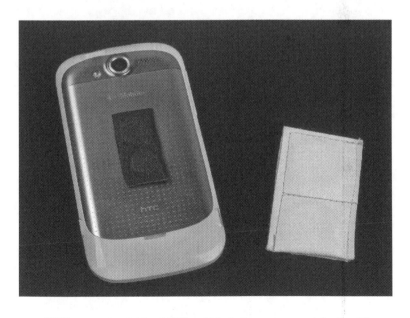

"What a great idea! Why didn't I come up with that?"

Slim Spurling

BACKGROUND OF THE PHONE RING SET

We all know how cordless phones, cell phones, and cell phone towers are hazardous to our health, yet we still use them. And some of us have an excessive dependency on these little gadgets.

When Katharina Spurling-Kaffl's friend Christine Schreier moved in to help her care for Slim in the summer of 2007, she had the idea of using rings on cordless phones to block EMF (electromagnetic field). She used her Virtual Con Pendulum to determine the best metal and plating to use, the size and type of ring, the placement of the rings in relationship to each other, and the type of material to use to encase them. Once the data was collected, Christine created the first Phone Ring Set.

She then experimented with the ring arrangement by making wireless and cell phone calls. Those who were called by an experimenter using a Phone Ring Set all reported a sense of calm and an opening of the heart chakra, along with relief of stress. Later, calls were made from wireless and cell phones without the Phone Ring Sets, and there were no reported changes. The experimenters themselves reported feeling more relaxed, and noticed a serene effect when placing calls on their wireless and cell phones.

PURPOSE OF THE PHONE RING SET

The Phone Ring Set is designed to help alleviate damage that may occur while frequently holding a cellular or cordless telephone to your ear for prolonged times. A recipient of a call will also find it to be a stress-relieving experience when speaking with someone who is calling with a Phone Ring Set on their phone.

DESCRIPTION OF THE PHONE RING SET

The set consists of one 1/8 Lost Cubit Ring and one 1/8 Sacred Cubit Ring sewn into a leather case, which measures 2½" x 1½". Because some cellular phones today are so compact, IX-EL, Inc. developed a smaller version of the Phone Ring Set, which measures 1½" x ¾". This smaller version, when tested, was still powerful enough to protect the user from most EMFs. It is important to note that the case and the rings should not be tampered with in any way. Each set of Phone Rings has an adhesive sheet attached so you can permanently stick it to the back of your phone. If you'd like to temporarily attach it to a phone, it is recommended to use a rubber band. This way, you can use it on your mobile phone, as well as your cordless phone.

APPLICATION OF THE PHONE RING SET

Place the Phone Ring Set on the back of a cordless or mobile phone to limit exposure to electromagnetic pollution that may harm body cells and damage DNA. It would be also perfect to place under your laptop, Kindle, or tablet.

Kinesiology is the scientific study of human movement and is the basis for this trial. We suggest you test your muscle strength by placing a Phone Ring Set under your laptop computer. You will likely find that your body is stronger when using the Phone Ring Set in this manner. The Phone Ring Set can also be placed under your laptop, iPad, tabloid, or Kindle with similar results.

FIELD REPORTS FROM RESEARCH ASSOCIATES

DR. OLDFIELD'S RESEARCH

"We became acquainted with Dr. Harry Oldfield in June of 2007. He came to our house to do a healing session on Slim. Previously, our friend Christine Schreier came up with the idea of a Phone Ring Set. We began to notice that some sensitive people around here felt better when we called them while using the Phone Ring Set on our phone.

"I contacted Dr. Oldfield to inquire as to whether he would be willing to do a blind study with one of our new creations. Dr. Oldfield agreed without knowing that I was calling from a telephone that had a Phone Ring Set attached. I asked him to take a picture of his associate, Evy, with Polycontrast Interference Photography (PIP) before a call I would make to her, then again during our call, and finally, during a second call.

"The first call was made from Colorado to England without the Phone Ring Set. Evy complained of feeling exhausted from a two-day training she had just completed and just wanted to go to bed. During the second call placed just minutes later, she said, "I don't know what you are doing, but I feel like partying, and my stress has disappeared." I could also hear Dr. Oldfield becoming very excited in the background, as he could see the immediate changes in her on his screen.

"The Light-Life™ Technology team continues to research the Phone Ring Set's potential!" *Katharina Spurling-Kaffl*

PHONE RINGS TESTED

"At the Heilpraktiker (naturopathic doctor) last week, I asked to test my cell phone with the rings on them. Result: the gauge went to about 20. It's notable that any reading below 50 is good for your system, or is an indication you need it!" *C.S., CA*

CELL PHONE IMPACT

"I am very happy to own a Phone Ring Set. I never knew how much impact my cell phone had on my body until I tried one of these. It feels as if it harmonizes the energy my phone emits, or neutralizes it so it does not travel into my body. This creates a much more pleasant and healthy experience for me when I talk on the phone or check my email on my BlackBerry. You can feel the difference! Thank you." *S.W., CO*

CHAPTER 19
Functional Art to Empower Your Life ~
The Light-Life™ Jewelry

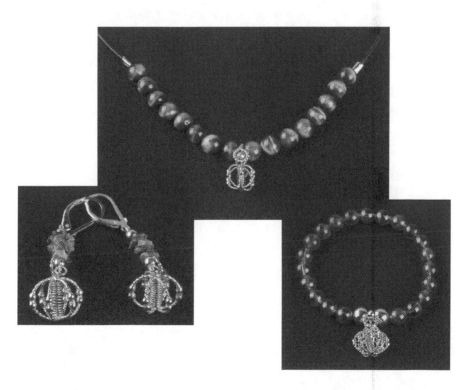

"The Mini Personal Harmonizer is just as effective as the standard size Personal Harmonizer, just gentler."

Audrey Cole

BACKGROUND OF MINI PERSONAL AND MINI PERSONAL UNITY HARMONIZER PENDANTS, EARRINGS AND BRACELETS

Katharina Spurling-Kaffl had a Tibetan Vajra cross pendant, also called a 'double Dorje,' which she was always very enamored of. She remembered that Slim once showed her a miniaturized version of the Personal Harmonizer, which his foster brother made. When she asked Slim why he didn't have them made, he responded it was because he didn't have a craftsman skilled in making this size. That is not the case today; Katharina's shop at IX-EL employs a very skilled craftswoman who, when showed the Vajra cross, became inspired. This young woman, always open to new challenges and very in-tune with Slim, made a Vajra cross pendant out of Mini Personal Harmonizers. This was the birth of the Light-Life jewelry made with Mini Personal Harmonizers in Sacred and Lost Cubit sizes, as well as the Unity Personal Harmonizer.

DESCRIPTION OF MINI PERSONAL AND MINI PERSONAL UNITY HARMONIZER PENDANTS, EARRINGS AND BRACELETS

The Mini Personal Harmonizers are half the size of the standard versions and made out of copper, and then plated with multiple layers of silver and gold. The necklaces and bracelets with one mini Personal Harmonizer come with a handmade clasp, which opens to allow the wearer to move the Harmonizer from one piece of jewelry to another.

The jewelry is also offered in different styles with gemstones. Quartz crystals seem to enhance the properties of the Harmonizer, while gemstone beads added to a piece of Harmonizer jewelry may enhance the gemstone's power. Swarovski crystals are sometimes added as decorative accents. On the IX-EL, Inc. website **www.LightLifeTechnology.com**, you will find many offerings of gemstone jewelry such as tiger eye, amethyst, and jade.

Earrings are made out of two Sacred Cubit Mini Personal Harmonizers. They come in two versions: slightly twisted, like the Standard Personal Harmonizer; and not twisted. Realizing that not everyone likes to wear earrings but may still desire the benefits this jewelry offers, Katharina came up with a great solution. She designed necklaces with two Sacred Cubit Personal Harmonizers evenly placed between precious gemstone beads.

PURPOSE OF MINI PERSONAL AND MINI PERSONAL UNITY HARMONIZER PENDANTS, EARRINGS, AND BRACELETS

According to several readings from clairvoyants on the jewelry, the earrings with Mini Harmonizers balance the chakras, align the matrix field around them, and gently raise the vibrations and frequencies into a place of perfect harmony. It is a melody, such that if you could hear it as music, would be a perfect harmonic tone. The diminutive size of the Mini Personal Harmonizers does not lessen their power. You will get the same benefit as from the larger Harmonizers.

When you are wearing Mini Harmonizer earrings, you are attuned to the balanced rhythm of the earth because of the elliptical energy surrounding the Harmonizer and intersecting with the logic of nature, your hormones, and your sleep patterns. You may find it creates a sense of well-being and brings you into a state of harmony. When you are in rhythm with nature, you naturally feel secure and safe. Use your focused intent to create desired results.

Apart from being very attractive pieces of art, the Mini Personal Harmonizers are recommended when you feel the need for extra protection of your energy field, keeping a clear mind in the midst of chaos, for calming yourself when you experience lot of stress, and when traveling, especially in airports or other crowded places like a mall or concert hall, the theater, and so forth.

APPLICATION OF MINI PERSONAL AND MINI PERSONAL UNITY HARMONIZER PENDANTS, EARRINGS, AND BRACELETS

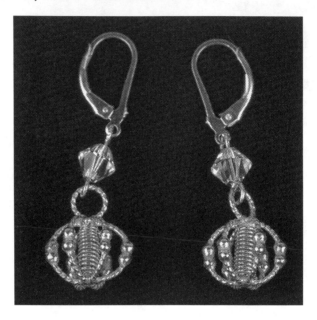

According to some very gifted clairvoyants and energy workers, wearing the earrings balances the brain hemispheres, as well as the chakras and whole body, down to the cellular level. Until you become accustomed to the energy from the earrings, you may want to wear them for just a few hours a day. Wearing the earrings with a Mini Personal Harmonizer necklace seems to provide an additional protection through creating a Merkaba field around the person.

When the Mini Personal Harmonizers are twisted, the energy of the earrings opens the heart and throat chakras and also activates the third eye. Another amazing benefit reported by some research associates is significant eyesight improvement. When wearing the earrings, a person should take off their glasses for an hour at a time, increasing time as progress permits. It should not be a strain on the eyes.

A Mini Harmonizer bracelet's effects depend upon which wrist the wearer chooses. Wearing the bracelet on the left wrist balances the female (inspiration) side. Worn on the right wrist, the bracelet balances out your male (action taker) side. If your energy is stuck and not moving, we suggest you wear the bracelet on your right wrist. If you feel uninspired, wear it on your left wrist. A female wanting to address her feminine side should wear the bracelet on her left wrist. If she wants to become stronger, more assertive, and courageous, she should wear it on her right wrist.

FIELD REPORTS FROM RESEARCH ASSOCIATES

SILVER PLATED EARRINGS WITH MINI PERSONAL HARMONIZER

"I'd like to share my experiences with the earrings I received for Valentine's Day. Although I am not normally a jewelry person, I do love the energy of the Light-Life Tools, and I was truly excited to receive the pair of earrings with the Mini Personal Harmonizers.

"In the beginning, I wore them only a few hours at a time. Now I use any "excuse" to wear them, and I must say, I feel more centered and calmer when I wear them. I noticed during especially difficult situations, they have been of great support. On top of that, people always notice them and remark how beautiful and unique they are. I am looking forward to receiving another elegant piece of your new jewelry." *D.C., MI*

EARRINGS AND EYE MASK REALIGN RODS AND CONES

"Haniel explained to me that the earrings and eye mask are helping to adjust and realign the rods and cones in my eyes, although they have a long way to go. Haniel also recommended that I use the eye mask for 20 minutes a day and Reiki my eyes while wearing the mask. She said that will also help give the recovery a boost. I can feel the energetic effect on my eyes while wearing the earrings, less so with the mask but that's okay as I'll take Haniel's word that it is assisting. I will continue to use them, while also saying my affirmations." *J.D., CO*

Earrings Help with Myopia

"I currently wear glasses, and have since I was 9 years old. I don't know off-hand my prescription, but it is under-corrected so that my eyes have to "work." My eyes are nearsighted (myopia). I take off my glasses as much as I can when I am home, on a walk, etc. I generally need them to drive, and I can sometimes read without them if I hold the article close enough.

"I wear the Harmonizer earrings draped over my ears using a glasses cord to hold them in place. They slip off of the screw-on clip frequently, causing me to be super aware of their presence. I wear them often, most of the day with and without the glasses. I say affirmations daily and Reiki my eyes everyday as well.

"It took about two weeks to notice much improvement. Then I began to notice that I could read the names of street signs much clearer than previously. I began to notice much more detail in nature; for example, I could see the leaves on the trees much clearer. I was not squinting to see street signs, and began to relax more while driving and in general. My vision appears to be improving, and I am very excited about the possibilities of this product.

"I have not been to the eye doctor but would love for him to see this and test my eyes. I am putting it off because I would like to experience just a little more improvement in my vision before my visit with him. He will be surprised and want to know what I have done! I will write more as I notice and keep you informed." *K.Z., CO*

Support for 2012 and Beyond ~
The Empowerment Ring

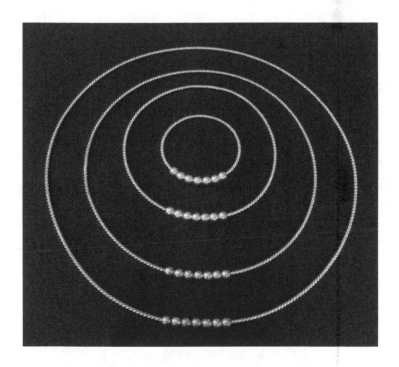

*"This ring completes the trinity of three
powerful cubit measurements."*

D.L.

BACKGROUND OF THE EMPOWERMENT RING

"It is my pleasure to announce the newest Light-Life™ Ring, which I am calling the **Empowerment Ring**. This ring is the final link in a trinity, as it is a newly revealed cubit measurement. The measurement was recently given to me by a gentleman who was in communication with Slim before his passing. Slim told him how to make the rings and took his promise not to make them commercially available. When Slim and this gentleman talked in 2006, we did not have the manufacturing capacity to make those rings. We were still manufacturing out of our three-car garage and our space was limited. This gentleman kept his promise and conveyed the information to me in 2011. We then made some prototypes and sent them to our research group for evaluation. The results were encouraging to go into production with this new measurement." *Katharina Spurling-Kaffl*

PURPOSE OF THE EMPOWERMENT RING

The purpose of the New Cubit Empowerment Ring is to support mental clarity and activity as well as enhance any healing processes, physically, mentally, and emotionally.

DESCRIPTION OF THE EMPOWERMENT RING

The Empowerment Ring is more than 10% larger than a Lost Cubit Ring and comes with seven beads. It is available in five sizes:

- ½ New Cubit copper, 24K gold plated
- 1 New Cubit copper, 24K gold plated
- 1½ New Cubit copper, 24K gold plated
- 2 New Cubit copper
- 3½ New Cubit copper

APPLICATION OF THE EMPOWERMENT RING

From Katharina Spurling-Kaffl: "Some of the feedback we've gotten suggests that intention is very important in using the Empowerment Ring. Beneficial results have been described as a calming of mental activity, increased clarity, and increased comprehension and understanding. When we shared our experiences with the gentleman who revealed the New Cubit measurement, he responded by saying, 'That is what my Spirit guides told me it would do. They also said it would bring completion.' We suggest experimenting with a combination of the three different cubit rings.

"Our impression is that all Light-Life Rings work multidimensionally. However, while we found that our Sacred Cubit Ring is best applied on the physical and the Lost Cubit Ring on the emotional, the Empowerment Ring appears to best support the mental."

FIELD REPORTS FROM RESEARCH ASSOCIATES

EMPOWERMENT RING SEEMS TO WORK WHERE IT'S NEEDED

"I have been working with the rings all week with my acupuncture clients. I have used both the Sacred Cubit and the New Cubit Empowerment Ring. I am especially enjoying working with the Empowerment Ring. I used it yesterday during an acupuncture session and found something quite interesting. I was working on my client's neck/shoulder and low back pain. I placed the ring over the needles on the neck/shoulder area first. When those were done, I removed them, then moved the ring to the low back area, which was still really active and not releasing. When I placed the ring on the low back, the whole area warmed up immediately. Tina felt like I had placed a heating blanket on her. When I removed the ring about 15 minutes later, the skin in the whole area was very warm to the touch (but not red like it would be with a heating blanket) and the warmth extended out further than the boundaries of the ring. I then used it around her umbilicus when I laid her on her back to activate her core energy. Like the shoulder area, that area did not feel appreciably warmer than the surrounding skin. I find this quite interesting. It is almost like the ring works in whatever way is most needed. Today Tina felt great, said it is the best and fastest she has ever responded to an acupuncture treatment (which I can attest to being true). I also used it last week on clients with the needles and had great results, with faster pain relief and immediate instead of delayed results. I am excited to keep "playing" with the rings and see what happens. I'll keep you posted. Also, I now have rings on my water softener tanks, refrigerator, and around my drinking water container. I can think of about a dozen more places to put them. I think you are right; you can't have too many rings!" *R.M., IN*

"Another note from R.M., IN: "I don't know if you know what radionics is, but using the ring on my antennae seriously cuts my broadcast times, which is nice, since that is the time-limiting factor in the process. Very powerful tool. I'll keep you posted."

Sound Healing and the Empowerment Ring

"I work with sound healing using Tuning Forks and Reiki. I began experimenting with two 1 cubit Empowerment Rings. At first I put them under the table in a Vesica Piscis pattern. Then two things happened that made me realize how powerful these rings are. First, my mother-in-law was having arm pain and numbness from her neck and face down to her hand. I immediately put her on a massage table and placed the two rings on her chest. I proceeded to use appropriate tuning forks along her arm. After about seven minutes, she reported that the feeling was coming back into her hands and the pain was softening in her upper arm. I continued the treatment for another 10 minutes and by then, her numbness was gone and the pain greatly diminished. I also used Ylang Ylang essential oil for her to inhale (it is known to help bring blood pressure down). She then went to the doctor who told her she was lucky, since it was a stroke. She is fine now.

"Another incident I noticed with the new rings: I was giving 20-minute demonstration sessions at a gathering. I knew that in 20 minutes I could give people a feeling for how powerful sound healing can be, but I didn't expect to see major things happen. I didn't have a massage table, so I couldn't put the rings under the table. I was using a bed, and I placed the rings on the front of my client's body, in a Vesica Piscis arrangement. I used Reiki symbols over the Empowerment Rings and sometimes put a Tibetan bowl in one of the rings.

"I was amazed that in more than three quarters of these sessions, the clients reported major improvements and many reported a complete disappearance of pain. Some reported a sense of feeling coming back to numb areas, and all reported a general happy humming of their bodies!!! I noticed that what usually took up to an hour to work happened in less than half that time. I was quite amazed and impressed with these magic rings!!" *H.I., CA*

TRANSMUTING MEMORIES WITH THE EMPOWERMENT RING

"I have been using the larger Empowerment Ring around my neck. The land we live on is full of earthbound spirits, and sometimes it messes with my head. I find myself reacting to thoughts that are not mine before I recognize their influence. The Empowerment Ring seems to keep the thoughts out of my head while I sleep and work.

"Additionally, the Empowerment Ring seems to be helping me process the abuse and the memories from my childhood as I acknowledge my father's passing and sort out the past at a deeper level. The Empowerment Ring seems to transmute painful memories past clearing and healing to learning, courage, and strength.

"Our African Grey Parrot loves the Empowerment Ring, too! If I lay on the floor with the ring around my neck, the ring pushes up and she likes to get on the pillow beside me, in the field, but not right in the ring. She snuggles with me and stays still instead of bugging me. It is a stunning difference. This is the mating and nesting season for birds, so for her to settle in like this and be sweet and quiet is very dramatic." *F.S., CO*

The Empowerment Ring was created and manufactured shortly before this book went to print in 2012. As time goes on, more field reports will be available. Please check our website **www.LightLifeTechnology.com** for continual updates and field reports.

NOTES:

Part III

A Toast to
Slim Spurling
1938-2007

*"...A remarkable man who dedicated his life to
restoring the health of the environment and mankind..."*

A friend and student

NOTES:

CHAPTER 21
Slim Spurling's Legacy ~
A World That Can Thrive

By Katharina Spurling-Kaffl

Slim and I shared a love of nature and its beauty, finding the truth in life, and the satisfaction of rewarding work. This was the beginning of an unexpected, but extraordinary life venture and partnership. In this lifetime, I came into Slim's life for several reasons, two of which were to give him the gift of freedom to explore and research his passion for truth and to experience unconditional love. By dedicating myself to the business, along with inspiring several new products, Slim gratefully became free to devote his time delving into his heart's desire.

Slim was a gifted teacher who would explain even the most difficult scientific material in a way that an ordinary audience could comprehend. I admired his ability to put people at ease and make them comfortable with the information he shared. On one of our first walks back from the workshop, Slim revealed that when he made the first Light-Life Ring, he had the insight that this ring could bring peace on Earth. I believe after reading this book, you will appreciate his statement and, undoubtedly, see the potential we have.

During our time together, Slim and I created many new products in the Light-Life™ Tools line. Our union continues still ~ for Slim's work will carry forward and expand under his guidance. Our years together helped prepare me for the responsibility of carrying on his legacy of the Light-Life Technology. Slim knew without question that I would continue our work with the same integrity and passion for healing our planet as we had devoted our lives to. He knew I would not make compromises when it came to the quality of the tools. Slim had confidence in my ability to discern between people who professed to be friends and those who genuinely cared. This faith was reassuring, as I was soon tested by acquaintances that were making and/or promoting counterfeit tools.

Slim's work lives on in the lives of our loyal customers, friends, and of course, our employees. Not only have we continued making the Light-Life Tools, but we've also created more products, all based on sacred geometry and quantum physics. My dedicated team and I are continuing Slim's research and the teaching of his Geobiology Workshops.

The beauty of the Light-Life Tools is that they're not stagnating; they are always expanding and adapting to changes on our planet and the earth's energies. I am open to the wisdom I get from the tools and will create new tools as they are shown to me. My intention is to organically present tools to people in the most expedient manner possible, yet in the most beneficial way. I am focused on offering only the highest quality tools.

Slim left an invaluable legacy and my hope is that you, the reader, are ignited by our vision. You can help spread the word and take the Light-Life Tools out in the world where they will have an enormous impact on people's lives, as well as the planet. After reading this book, I am sure you understand now there are no limits to their applications.

My vision is that the Light-Life Tools become a household name, be an essential part in every first aid kit, and are used to significantly reduce environmental pollution. I'd like to see people everywhere have at least one Light-Life Ring in their arsenal. A Harmonizer in every community to bring harmony, clean the air, and counteract severe weather conditions would be ideal. Used alone or in combination with other technology, these tools enhance positive outcomes for many and inspire harmony. We have the technology to change the face of this planet for the better. Let's do it!

Please make sure to visit our website **LightLifeTechnology.com** often to get updates on our latest developments. Sign up for the newsletter to stay in communication and to learn about future workshops and webinars.

PART IV
Resources

NOTES:

Light-Life™ Ring Size & Dimension Chart

SIZE	DIMENSION " = inches cm = centimeter	COPPER	AVAILABLE IN:		
			COPPER 24K GOLD PLATED	STERLING SILVER	STERLING SILVER, 24K GOLD PLATED
½ Sacred Cubit	3.5"/8.9cm	*	*B3	*B2	
½ Lost Cubit	4.0"/10.2cm	*	*B3		*B2
½ New Cubit	4.2"/10.8cm		*B7		
1 Sacred Cubit	6.5"/16.5cm	*	*B3	*B2	*B2
1 Lost Cubit	7.5"/19.1cm	*	*B3	*B2	
1 Sacred Cubit heavy no beads	6.0"/15.2cm		*		
1 Lost Cubit heavy no beads	7.0"/17.8cm		*		
1 New Cubit	8.5"/21.6cm		*B7		
1½ Sacred Cubit	10.0"/25.4cm	*B3	*B3	*B2	*B2
1½ Lost Cubit	11.2"/28.4cm	*B3	*B3		
1½ Sacred Cubit heavy no beads	9.7"/24.6cm	*	*		
1½ Lost Cubit heavy no beads	11.0"/27.9cm	*	*		
1½ New Cubit	12.7"/32.3cm		*B7		
2 Sacred Cubit	13.2"/33.5cm	*B5	*B5		
2 Sacred Cubit heavy no beads	13.0"/33.0cm	*	*		
2 Lost Cubit	15.0"/38.1cm	*B5			
2 Lost Cubit heavy no beads	14.7"/37.3cm	*	*		
2 New Cubit	17.0"/43.2cm	*B7			
3½ Sacred Cubit	23.5"/59.7cm	*B5			
3½ Sacred Cubit heavy	23.0"/58.4cm	*B5			
3½ Lost Cubit	26.2"/66.5cm	*B5			
3½ Lost Cubit heavy	26.0"/66.0cm	*B5			
3½ New Cubit	30.0"/76.2cm	*B7			
		B2 = Contains 2 Beads B3 = Contains 3 Beads B4 = Contains 4 Beads B5 = Contains 5 Beads B7 = Contains 7 Beads			

This configuration, used in conjunction with an Agricultural Harmonizer, has been successful in stopping flooding in New Hampshire, halting severe thunderstorms in Tennessee, and improving overall weather conditions in Alaska. Please feel free to copy this for your personal use.

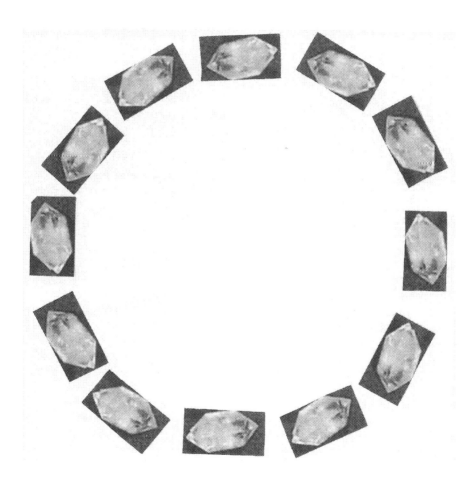

Appendix B
Media Products

Dowsing & Light-Life™ Tools DVD

This DVD is for the beginning student wishing to familiarize him or herself with the art of dowsing. Slim Spurling teaches how to work with earth energies through dowsing. Learn how to locate and neutralize the Hartmann Grid, geopathic zones, and other types of geopathic stress.

Interview with Alan Steinfeld DVD

This DVD is a great opportunity to "meet" Slim Spurling and learn about some of the tools and his vision.

Environmental Clearing CD

The Environmental Clearing CD is a recording of the molecular frequencies of water, the Universal Solvent, and the prime substance required by all living things. An examination of this audio by electronic spectrum analyzer yields a random appearing list of individual frequencies ranging from zero to over 30,000 Hz. Many of the frequencies repeat at irregular intervals, which has given rise to the idea that the whole set of frequencies may be an algorithm, possibly even the algorithm of life itself.

Environmental observations, when these frequencies are coupled with the Harmonizer's energy field, are of a great increase in the vitality of plants and animals within the Harmonizer's range of effect. This can vary from 15 to 65 miles in radius. Just as living organisms change water, air and minerals from the soil into various molecules within the organism, the Harmonizer's energy field appears to break down toxins in the environment into neutral or non-toxic substances; possibly into life sustaining substances. The proliferation of plant growth and the ability of soils to produce a 30 to 100% increase in yield under severe drought conditions are among the observed effects noted. (See website under

Field Reports.) Bio-assays of bacteria laden waters show a sharp decline in infectious bacteria, and Dinoflagellates, and toxic algae. Certain field crops become dramatically healthier and, consequently, do not attract insects.

Grandmother's Drum CD

The Grandmother's Drum frequency is more advanced and should be used with caution. It is meant to take the user into a deep meditation. Avoid driving and other activities while listening to this recording. The recorded frequencies of Grandmother's Drum are derived from the recorded frequencies scanned with Molecular Frequency Scanner of the whole environment following the first Air Pollution Clearing event conducted in Denver on 18 March 1994. Sample scans were taken for short periods every fifteen minutes from 2 pm until 7 pm. The frequencies were then run through a Fourier analysis software program. The resulting graphic was a smooth curve from high amplitude to low, and even negative amplitude. It could be represented as a long, drawn out sigh of relief from the environment, as--- OOOOOHHHHHHhhhhhhhhhHHHHhhhh::::::......... in fact, inaudible, but demonstrating a reduction of the amount of chaos in the environment from high to zero. Chaos equals resistance = heat = pain. Absence of chaos = conductivity = coolness = no pain = superconductivity.

Using the Grandmother's Drum CD with the Harmonizer seems to push the environment toward calmness and "flowingness." On a mental level, when listened to with earphones or on low volume on a stereo, the body moves into a very relaxed state where even long held subconscious tensions let go. Creativity seems to go into high gear after a few short hours of listening. The CD program is deliberately made short because of its extraordinarily powerful effects. Once through the recording every hour for a day is about as much creativity as one can tolerate. The mental processes speed up and ideas seem to come out of the blue, often accompanied by mental pictures embodying the ideas. Clarity is also enhanced. Please make very careful observations of the indoor and outdoor environments before, during, and after using the CD. Unusual cloud patterns may appear, and other changes in light quality and sound quality may become evident to various senses.

King's Chamber Resonance CD

The King's Chamber Resonance CD was produced by Hans Becker as a 'brain balancer' to enable integration of the right and left hemispheres, resulting in profound elevation of awareness and creativity. Think of what you would like to manifest while meditating with this CD and listening on earphones.

Appendix C
Glossary

BTS: Abbreviation for Beyond the Sky Light-Life™ Rings.

Counterfeit Tools: Tools that look like the original Slim Spurling Light-Life™ Tools or very similar, however, they are not manufactured by Slim Spurling or IX-EL, Inc. The original Slim Spurling Light-Life™ Tools have been manufactured since 1991, and only Katharina Spurling-Kaffl has permission from Slim Spurling to do so. To ensure you have an original Light-Life™ Tool, please check the distributor list found on the websites of **www.LightLifeTechnology.com** and **www.SlimSpurling.com**.

Cubit: An ancient unit of linear measure.

Dowsing: A technique of communication used to translate the information between the conscious and subconscious mind through the use of an instrument, such as a pendulum or dowsing rod.

Dowsing Tools: Instruments used for dowsing include the pendulum, L-Rod, Y-Rod, and Bobber.

Dissonance: When two waves vibrating at different frequencies meet, they create chaos.

Earth Energies: Earth energies occur naturally all over the planet, forming a web-like grid around, through, and above the earth. These earth energies can be both positive and negative, or referred to as beneficial, i.e., Ley Lines, and detrimental, i.e., geopathic stress lines, in their impact on those that live and work in or near them.

Electromagnetic Spectrum: The range of frequencies of electromagnetic waves which include radio, infrared, visible light, ultraviolet, X-ray, and gamma ray waves.

ELF: Extremely Low Frequency.

EMF: Electromagnetic fields are caused by power lines, home wiring, airport and military radar, substations, transformers, cell phones and cell phone towers, computers, and appliances.

Entrainment: When two or more oscillating objects lock into a cycle so they are synchronized in their vibrations.

Frequency: Rate of vibration.

Geobiology: The study of the interactions of life with the physical earth.

Geopathic Stress: The name given to natural or man-made energies emanating from the earth which are detrimental to human health as well as animal and plant health.

Hartmann Grid: Earth energy lines, magnetic in nature, creating an invisible grid over the surface of the earth, oriented to the earth's magnetic field. Direction of flow: south north and west east. These lines can adversely affect living organisms, especially at lines of intersection.

Ley Lines: Part of the earth's beneficial energy system, an invisible network of straight lines connecting one power site to another, which can extend hundreds of miles.

Light-Life™ Technology: Is a cutting edge technology based on the blending of ancient and modern science and knowledge.

Lost Cubit: A linear measurement, discovered by Hans Becker, also called the "forbidden, hidden, or Becker cubit," filling a harmonic gap between the established Sacred and Royal Cubits. The one Lost Cubit vibrates at the frequency of 177 MHz.

Merkaba: A counter-rotating field of light generated from the spinning of specific geometric forms that simultaneously affects one's spirit and body. It is a vehicle that can aid mind, body, and spirit to access and experience other planes of reality or potentials of life.

Neter: The ancient measurements known of length.

New Cubit: A final link in a trinity of cubit measurements, the New Cubit is a recently revealed measurement given to Katharina Spurling-Kaffl by a gentleman who was in communication with Slim before his passing.

Orte der Kraft: locations or sites endowed with an energy, a force, a strength.

Paradigm: An example that serves as a pattern or model for something, especially one that forms the basis of a methodology or theory.

Plating: Plating is the process of applying a thin coat or plate of a selected metal to a conductive surface.

Potentized: A Light-Life™ Ring increases the available energy in the water instantaneously.

Psychotronic: The ability to control the physical world with your mind.

Resonance: An effect brought on by sympathetic vibration between two compatible vibratory processes.

Sacred Cubit: An ancient measurement found at the Great Pyramid of Giza carved in stone just above the entrance to the King's Chamber. The one Sacred Cubit vibrates at the frequency of 144 MHz.

Sacred Geometry: The way Spirit integrates into matter through geometric form, structure, and design.

Scalar Energy: Electromagnetic waves that exist only in the vacuum of empty space.

Schumann Resonance: Heartbeat of the earth, the frequency of the earth in the ELF range (extremely low frequency) of the earth's total electromagnetic spectrum.

Sensitives: Those with clairvoyant abilities being able to see beyond the ordinary realm of perception.

Superconductivity: The flow of electric current without resistance in certain metals, alloys, and ceramics at temperatures near absolute zero.

Tensor: A term from quantum physics; is an energy field that supports matter, for example, the energy field which supports a soap bubble on a bubble wand.

Toroid: Geometric shape. For example, a donut shape.

Torus: Is the surface area of a toroid, and the toroid is the form encased by a torus. It is a sphere shape that curves inward on top and bottom, having a hole in the center.

Vesica Piscis: Pointed oval shape created when two circles of the same size intersect by touching the center of the circumference of each other.

Vibration: An oscillating movement in one direction, then back again in the opposite direction.

References

Slim Spurling
www.SlimSpurling.com

IX-EL, Inc.
3182 Tipple Parkway, Erie, CO 80516
1-877-239-0211
www.IX-EL.com

IX-EL International GmbH
Am Kirchsteig 29, D-86928 Hofstetten, GERMANY
(49) 08196-934-325
www.IXELGmbH.com
info@IXELGmbH.com

Susan Anderson
www.seedsforchangewellness.com

American Society of Dowsers
www.dowsers.org
asd@dowsers.org

Aranya
Light Life Tools UK
www.lightlifetools.co.uk
mail@lightlifetools.co.uk

Tana Blackmore, founder of Sacred Ground International
www.sacredgroundintl.org
406-245-6070

Audrey Cole
www.AAHaniel.com

Anthony Cowan is a licensed Pranic Healing practitioner in Sarasota, Florida. Anthony works on people, animals, properties, and the environment.
anthonyprana@gmail.com
941-284-0153

Ellie Drew
www.elliedrew.com

Joyce Frost
Oakdale, CA
joanarc@sbcglobal.net
209-845-1313

Briar Hill Holistics & Gift - Beth Hampel
29583 North Gossell Road, Wauconda, IL 60084
847-526-3681

Sherry Houck
1306 Via Robles, Santa Fe, NM 87501
noegrets@comcast.net
505-989-4691

Virginia Houck, LMT
36 Tattersall Lane, Albany, NY 12205
wellnessessentials@msn.com
518-869-6413

Heidi Irgens
www.energease.com

Michael W. Kaffl
Am Kirchsteig 29, D-86928 Hofstetten, GERMANY
(49) 08196-9989-486
www.InnovativeProdukte.com
innovapro@t-online.de

Dr. Lenny Lee Kloepper
www.DocLenny.com
719-371-3954

Judy Lavine
Medical Intuitive ~ Healer ~ Shaman
www.judylavine.com

Life Technology™
Transformational Technology For Mind Body And Soul™
www.lifetechnology.com
lifetech@lifetechnology.com

Marilyn Melvin ~ Air, Water & Wellness
503-524-4862

Dr. Harry Oldfield
www.electrocrystal.com

Christine Schreier
www.ThePuppenstube.com

West Coast Dowsers
www.dowserswestcoast.org
dowserina@earthlink.net

Sam Zeiger
New York, NY
www.bluelightfloatation.com

ACKNOWLEDGEMENTS

Slim and I shared a heartfelt desire to help heal our planet and everyone living on it. I could not have carried on with our work without our dedicated employees in the U.S. and Germany, whose support has been invaluable to me. They take great pride in maintaining the high quality of the tools and upholding our reputation of providing exceptional customer service. The commitment of my shop craftsmen to manufacture genuine products, with the integrity Slim intended, continues to this day. Their loyalty is a blessing to me.

My brother, Michael Kaffl, was my introduction to Slim, and I am forever grateful to him. Michael was responsible for bringing Slim to Germany. He studied with Slim, and his understanding of the science of the tools is of great value to me. I can always count on Michael for his unwavering loyalty and advice.

My assistant, Diane Covington, took on the challenge of editing this book at a time when she was just learning about the tools. Her perseverance and pronounced skills of the English language helped shape this book and ready it for publication. It was fun working with her and improving my English in the process!

To Richard Nickol and my other esteemed editors whose editing contributions were invaluable, I count myself fortunate to have benefitted from your expertise.

I would like to acknowledge my friend Sherry Houck, who volunteered endless hours transcribing recordings of Slim's talks. I am very grateful for her labor of love and all the time she generously gave to bring Slim's words to you.

Rebekka Potter with iUniverse and Triona O'Donoghue with KillerCovers. com exhibited nothing but professionalism and competence in guiding us through the maze of self-publishing. The swift communication they both consistently provided made this project manageable.

I want to express my sincere appreciation to all those friends who helped me reconnect with Slim and gave me encouragement and empowerment when I most needed it.

To my Mastermind Group ~ Deborah Johnson, Denise Stillman, and Diana Sheridan ~ whose encouragement and professional opinions helped guide me through the process of bringing this book to fruition ~ thank you ladies.

Kudos to my coach, Debbie DeVoe, who was here from the very beginning of this project and gave me inspiration and guidance, as well as my coach, Will Mattox, who came into my life during the final stage of the book and offered invaluable suggestions.

Thank you to all our friends and associates who contributed in many different ways to support our work and spread the Light-Life™ Technology worldwide. I also want to give credit to those who kindly sent in their field reports to make the content more tangible and valuable to you, the reader. Their candid encounters with the tools can be used as a guide to lead you to an improved quality of life.

I thank you, the reader, who has shown your commitment for a clean planet by incorporating the tools in your daily life. You are the reason we persevere!

And last, but not least, I am forever grateful for Slim's genius and his dedication to find remedies for environmental pollution, and to give people the tools to heal themselves. It is he who took me on the most rewarding journey of my life and opened my eyes to so many possibilities I was not consciously aware of.

Katharina Spurling-Kaffl

BIBLIOGRAPHY

WORKS CITED

American Society of Dowsers. N.p., n.d. Web. 2 Apr. 2010. <http://www.dowsers.org/index.htm>.

Anderson, Scott. "Geobiology: A New Frontier." *Seeds for Change Wellness.* Susan Anderson, Sept. 2008. Web. 19 Mar. 2010. <http://www.seedsforchangewellness.com/ArticleGeobiologyTheNewFrontier.html>.

Baldwin, H W. "Dowsers Detect Enemy's Tunnel." *New York Times* 13 Oct. 1967: 17. Print.

Becker, Robert. *Cross Currents.* New York: Penguin, 1990. Print.

Becker, Robert, and Gary Selden. *The Body Electric: Electromagnetism and the Foundation of Life.* New York: Morrow, 1985. Print.

Bucher, Jay L. The Metrology Handbook. Milwaukee: William A. Tony, 2004. Print.

Burke, Dee, and Kenneth Burke. "Slim Spurling and His Light-Life Tools." *The Leading Edge* 1997: n. pag. Web. 20 Mar. 2010. <http://www.4dshift.com/back/may98.htm>.

- - -. "Technology to Clean the Planet." *Mind Tools Graphics.* N.p., n.d. Web. 17 Apr. 2010. <http://www.mindtoolsgraphics. com/ LoreRainbow/ Dousing4GeoStress.htm>.

Chandler, Wayne B. Ancient Future: The Teachings and Prophetic Wisdom of the Seven Hermetic Laws of Ancient Egypt. Atlanta: Penguin Putnam, 1999. Print.

Donlan, Joseph E. *Ordaining Reality in Brief: The Shortcut to Your Future.* Boca Raton, FL: Universal, 2009. Print.

Dossey, Barbara Montgomery, and Lynn Keegan. *Holistic Nursing: A Handbook of Practice.* Sudbury, MA: Jones and Bartlett, 2009. Print.

Einstein, Albert. "Correspondence between Herman E. Peisach and Albert Einstein." *Dowsing Works.* International Society of Dowsers, n.d. Web. 21 Mar. 2010. <http://dowsingworks.com/ einstein.html>.

Farmer, Steven D. *Earth Magic: Ancient Shamanic Wisdom for Healing Yourself, Others, and the Planet.* N.p.: Hay, 2009. Print.

Geobiology- Dowsing & Light-Life™ Tools. 2007. IX-EL, Inc. DVD.

"How Electromagnetic Radiation Becomes Your Invisible Killer." *Alternative-Magnetic-Therapy.* N.p., n.d. Web. 21 Mar. 2010. <http:// www.alternative-magnetic-therapy.com/electromagnetic-radiation. html>.

Howells, J. Harvey. *Dowsing for Everyone.* 1982

"Lengths." Beyond Energy Healing. Regina Hampton, n.d. Web. 4 May 2010. <http://www.beyondenergyhealing.com/sc_lenghts.shtml>.

Light-Life™ Technology. N.p., n.d. Web. 2 Apr. 2010. <http://**www. lightlifetechnology.com**/>.

Mid-Atlantic Geomancy. Sig Lonegren, n.d. Web. 10 Apr. 2010. <http:// www.geomancy.org/dowsing/ l-rods/#index.php>.

Morgan, Bill. *Scalar Energy – A Completely New World is Possible.*

Moser, Sabina. "Interview with Slim Spurling." Munich, Germany 2006.

Nielsen, Greg, and Joseph Polanksy. *Pendulum Power: A Mystery You Can See, A Power You Can Feel.* Vermont: Destiny, 1997. Print.

"Plating." Wikipedia. N.p., 28 Apr. 2010. Web. 3 May 2010. <http://en.wikipedia.org/wiki/Plating>.

Ross, T E, and Richard Wright. *The Divining Mind: A Guide to Dowsing and Self-Awareness.* Vermont: Destiny, 1990. Print.

Seaward, Brian Luke. *Managing Stress: Principles and Strategies for Health and Well Being, Volume 1.* Sudbury, MA: Jones and Bartlett, 2006. Print.

Slim Spurling: Interview with Alan Steinfeld. 2006. IX-EL, Inc. DVD.

Slim Spurling's Universe: Introduction and Application of the Light-Life™ Tools. 2004. IX-EL Publishing LLC. DVD.

Spurling, Slim. "The Acu-Vac Coils." *Conscious Mind Journal.* N.p., Apr. 2007. Web. 12 Apr. 2010. <http://www.consciousmindjournal.com/Articles/2007-04-01/THE-ACU-VAC-COILS.cfm>.

- - -. "The Light-Life™ Rings." *Conscious Mind Journal.* N.p., Mar. 2007. Web. 13 Apr. 2010. <http://www.consciousmindjournal.com/Articles/2007-03-01/The-Light-Life-Rings.cfm>.

- - -. "Slim's Technical Information." *MZ Alchemist Oils.* N.p., 4 May 2000. Web. 12 Apr. 2010. <http://www.4dshift.com/ products/ slimtechnical. htm>.

Tom, Lynch. Superconductivity for Teachers and High School and Middle School Students. cefa.fsu.edu. N.p., 2003. Web. 7 May 2010. <www.cefa.fsu.edu/Superconductivity for Teachers Aug. 2009. Final. ppt>.Power Point Presentation

Wheeler, John Archibald. *Geometrodynamics*. New York: Academic, 1962. Print.

Wilson, Jim. "Finding Water With A Forked Stick May Not Be A Hoax." *Popular Mechanics* Nov. 1998: n. pag. Print.

- - -. "Finding Water With A Forked Stick May Not Be A Hoax." *Popular Mechanics* Nov. 1998: n. pag. Web. 1 Apr. 2010.<http:// www. popularmechanics.com/science/research/1281661.html>.

INDEX